THE MOST EFFECTIVE WAYS TO
TAKE BACK YOUR BACK

BETH B. MURINSON, M.D., PH.D.

Director of Pain Education, Department of Neurology, Johns Hopkins School of Medicine

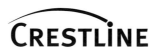

CRESTLINE

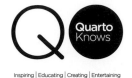

Inspiring | Educating | Creating | Entertaining

Brimming with creative inspiration, how-to projects, and useful information to enrich your everyday life, Quarto Knows is a favorite destination for those pursuing their interests and passions. Visit our site and dig deeper with our books into your area of interest: Quarto Creates, Quarto Cooks, Quarto Homes, Quarto Lives, Quarto Drives, Quarto Explores, Quarto Gifts, or Quarto Kids.

Text © 2011 Beth B. Murinson, M.S., M.D., Ph.D.

This edition published in 2018 by Crestline,
an imprint of The Quarto Group
142 West 36th Street, 4th Floor
New York, NY 10018 USA
T (212) 779-4972 F (212) 779-6058
www.QuartoKnows.com

First published in the USA in 2011 by Fair Winds Press,
an imprint of The Quarto Group, 100 Cummings Center,
Suite 265D, Beverly, MA 01915-6101

10 9 8 7 6 5 4 3 2 1

Crestline titles are also available at discount for retail, wholesale, promotional, and bulk purchase. For details, contact the Special Sales Manager by email at specialsales@quarto.com or by mail at The Quarto Group, Attn: Special Sales Manager, 401 Second Avenue North, Suite 310, Minneapolis, MN 55401, USA.

ISBN-13: 978-0-7858-3590-5

Printed and bound in China

Book Design: Kathie Alexander
Layout: Kathie Alexander
Illustrator: Robert Brandt

The information in this book is for educational purposes only. It is not intended to replace the advice of a physician or medical practitioner. Please see your health-care provider before beginning any new health program.

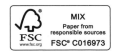

To Sasha,

מצתי אתה שאהבת נפשי

CONTENTS

2 | Getting Better, Getting Stronger /166

Preface: Not All Back Pain Is Alike

It is obvious to most people that back pain doesn't happen to every person in exactly the same way. Yet much of today's medical literature fails to guide back pain sufferers and the clinicians who care for them through the manifold challenges of recovering from acute back injury and chronic back pain. The most worrisome clinical reports lump all back pain together, urging physicians to attribute a patient's "complaints" to generic low back pain unless certain "red flags" are identified. Some reports unwisely assume that all conservative treatments are the same and should be equally potent against all forms of back pain. It seems that back pain research is dominated by those who have minimal direct contact with people actually suffering from back pain. This treat-all-back-pain-alike approach deeply disregards the need to apply the best of modern medicine to alleviate the profound suffering caused by specific back problems.

The forces driving the oversimplification of back pain care are system-wide. There are pressures from businesses to minimize back-related absences from work; from ambitious office managers to reduce the duration of medical visits; from pharmaceutical companies to expand the profits from pain-relieving medications; and from insurers who must otherwise reimburse workers for time spent recovering from injury. The overlapping interests of these various groups have fostered the creation of "educational symposia." These symposia promote a single perspective on back-injury science showcasing highly-paid experts who perpetuate the notion that the most back pain episodes cannot be precisely diagnosed. They tell the clinicians in attendance that attempting to do so is a waste of valuable clinical effort. The simplistic ideas that pain killers are the only proven treatment, and that the only non-pharmacological intervention that a sensible doctor can make is to urge patients to continue activity at normal levels are the take-home messages. To make matters worse, by oversimplifying the effects of gender on pain processing, these educational symposia often reinforce stereotypes that limit women's access to care.

It is clear from my clinical practice, personal experience, and speaking to people around the country that this approach to back care fails the Reality Test: Insisting that all back pain is the same just doesn't make sense. The spine is a complex structure; in fact, it is a bio-engineering miracle. Composed of bones, ligaments, nerves, and muscles all working together, the spine allows us to stand upright with the advantages of speedy locomotion and sophisticated hand functions. We would never give up the benefits we enjoy from walking upright. And so, each of us must come to terms with the consequences of an upright posture. Routine exercise and diet are not enough; people need enhanced knowledge of their backs and a deeper understanding of how to build a reservoir of strength and attain freedom from pain-imposed limitations.

This book was created as an open guide for people currently suffering from back pain due to non-operable back injury. The purpose was to bring together top science on back pain with both bona fide and evolving approaches to recovering from back injury. Despite hitting some serious notes here in the introduction, the book itself maintains a friendly, optimistic tone. This is because we know that maintaining a positive, proactive stance really does promote better health outcomes. Remind yourself daily that the glass is not only "half full," it is half full of a wonderful life-giving liquid with dozens of health benefits. Drink up and go get another! It is my vision that in reading this book, you will find help and a wealth of useful information. You will reinforce existing good habits and get inspired to try new back-healthy activities. This book is the best of everything that I could know, learn, and find to guide people in getting better from back injury. It is here to speed your journey toward a long and happy life without back pain.

Introduction: How to Use This Book

Because your back is central to everything you do, sitting, standing, walking, and even lying down can be problematic when pain strikes. If you have back pain when sitting, it is likely that working at a desk, eating at a dinner table, and driving are next to impossible. Having back pain when standing or walking puts participation in everyday life out of reach. And back pain when lying down is a prescription for insomnia without the aid of powerful drugs. Ring a bell? You may be experiencing problems similar to these or have an important person in your life who suffers from back pain. Whatever your reason for purchasing this book, you are in the right place. This book is written to guide you, your family, and your friends on the journey to a healthy back.

Take Back Your Back is a synthesis of tested methods for improving back pain. The difficult part of this therapy is that it requires an investment of time and energy, by you as well as your support team: family, friends, doctors, nurses, physical therapists, and co-workers. Knowing what to do when back pain is severe will save hours of frustration and disappointment. Even when there is no quick fix, many things can be done to alleviate acute back pain and speed a return to function. I sometimes explain these methods to patients using the name Aggressive Conservative Therapy, but in reality it is most fundamentally about making peace with your back. Repairing, restoring, nurturing, cultivating, strengthening, building, and ultimately healthy enjoyment of the back are all part of this approach.

In Part I, I describe the major causes of back pain, from muscle-related problems to coccydynia. Many structures in the back can be injured and result in pain. There are 12 thoracic vertebrae, 5 lumbar vertebrae, sacral bones, a tailbone or coccyx, over 20 discs, dozens of facet joints, scores of ligaments, 44 nerve roots, many muscles, and hundreds of nerve branches. When several of these structures are injured at the same time, as often happens with a trauma to the back, the pain is amplified. So it's often very difficult to identify the exact source of a problem. This book will help you identify your pain and work with your doctor to receive better care.

To make the book truly accessible, I have put the diagnosis and prescriptions for each condition first, followed by information about diagnostic tests and detailed explanations. *Take Back Your Back* is a reference book. I don't expect you to read every page! Look at the table of contents to find the kind of pain you're experiencing, and go directly to that chapter. Part II contains information about preventing and treating back pain, with chapters on exercise, ergonomics, and nutrition.

IT'S VITAL TO KEEP YOUR OWN RECORDS

I would like to emphasize the importance of keeping records about your health and back problem that you experience. Our society is mobile and dynamic; most Americans live away from their hometowns. In most places, the retention of "permanent" medical records is controlled by law, and after a certain period of inactivity, your doctor may simply discard the records pertaining to your medical condition. If this happens, you won't be able to go back and get your old records; they will no longer exist. Here's why keeping personal medical records is so important:

- Communicating with new providers about your problem will be easier
- Having an accurate medical history can prevent medical errors
- Reviewing records is a great way to learn more about your condition

I suggest making short- and long-term goals for your record keeping:

SHORT-TERM GOAL: Make a one-page health summary that lists your doctors, medicines, and health conditions. Include a short timeline of events relating to your major health problems. If your back pain arises from a specific injury, note that date and others relevant to your treatment course. Keep this one-page summary up to date, carry it with you at all times, and make a copy for your doctor and for your close ones. Also, make sure that any images of your back are kept with your records.

LONG-TERM GOAL: Make and maintain a health file that includes notes from doctor visits, lab reports, imaging reports, images on disc or film, a pain calendar or symptom diary, and notes from physical therapy. It's a good idea to keep your file or diary organized by record type, and arrange it in chronological fashion. Also, because X-rays, MRIs, and other imaging representations are pictures of a single point in time, make sure you keep copies of any images taken of your back in chronological files.

You are your own best advocate for better health care. Read on to identify and relieve your back pain, and keep those records handy for recurring problems. Your back is central to everything you do, and keeping it healthy and strong is fundamental to living well.

PART 1

Diagnose and Relieve Your Back Pain

CHAPTER 1

Muscle-Related Back Pain

Muscle injury and overuse is often the culprit.

Reduce inflammation and shift activities to avoid re-injury.

the DIAGNOSIS

> **Do you have pain located on one side of the spine?**

> **Does your pain stay focused in the back without radiating into the leg or another part of the body?**

Pain that is focused on one side of the back and does not radiate into the leg, groin, or torso is often due to muscle injury. Most typically, this type of back pain will follow a specific strain or stress to the muscle. It's often simply a case of "over-doing it," whether from lifting something a little too heavy, twisting around with the body for something just out of reach, or being overly aggressive with weekend sports. The large muscles on either side of the spine are prone to athletic injury, while the smaller muscles closer to the spine can be damaged by twisting movements.

Back muscle pain often has a burning quality, but when intense, it can be sharply painful and abruptly limit normal movement. One way to test for muscle pain is by first getting into a comfortable position. Now, gently start to initiate movement in a direction that you know will bring out your back pain. If your back pain is located off center (not directly over the spine) and does not radiate down the leg, into the groin, or around to the front of the body, you may have a back muscle injury, and this is the chapter for you.

If this does not describe your back pain, consider alternatives by reading the next chapter on radiating back pain and consulting a qualified health professional.

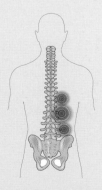

the PRESCRIPTION

To promote healing of your injured muscles, you'll need to reduce inflammation and prevent re-injury. Once inflammation and the potential for re-injury are under control, your muscles will stop hurting so terribly and healing will begin.

If you have a back muscle injury (sometimes referred to as *back muscle strain*):
- Your doctor may recommend physical therapy, especially if it seems that your back strain is not getting better on its own or if the problem keeps occurring.
- Your doctor may encourage you to stay active after a couple of days of taking it easy.
- Your doctor will likely encourage you to continue working and may provide a recommendation for pain medication to get you through this episode of pain.

Lifestyle changes for your back are going to be essential in plotting your course toward permanent recovery from a back muscle injury and pain. You'll need to focus on stretching, strengthening, and symmetry. But first, you've got to get the pain under control. I call this "back muscle First Aid," and outline the program in this chapter.

Medications are also part of getting better after muscle injury. Your healthcare provider may advise you about particular medications and will want to know what you've been taking at home. Make sure to follow recommended guidelines for taking medications and never, ever take someone else's prescription pain medicine.

The Treatment

Reducing inflammation is essential when you have a sudden, severe muscle pain problem. But if you are having persistent back pain that your doctor says is caused by muscle problems, chances are that you are chronically re-injuring your back muscles. The following strategies will begin to break this painful cycle.

Phase 1: How Do You Spell Relief? RICE-M

The best therapies for acute muscle strain are Rest, Ice, Compression, Elevation, and (anti-inflammatory) Medication. These treatments, best used in combination, are remembered with the acronym RICE-M. Picture a young athlete with a muscle strain, sitting on a table in the treatment room (Rest), ice pack bound in place with an elastic bandage (Ice and Compression), with the leg or arm propped up on a block (Elevation), being instructed by the trainer to take some food before each dose of ibuprofen tablets (Medication). All of these treatment components play an important role in preventing a worsening of the injury and speeding the return to function.

R IS FOR REST

Rest is a special challenge when the back is involved. We depend heavily on our backs for all parts of everyday life. Sitting, walking, standing, lifting the groceries, bending down to pick up a child or pet; the things we do range from mildly stressful on the back to extremely demanding. One of the worst offenders for back stress is housework, that burden of daily life that weighs upon those of us not yet admitted to the jet set. Some housework is undoubtedly benign for the back. Even though it gets a bad rap, cleaning windows can offer healthy opportunities for stretching and strengthening the arm muscles and upper back.

In the acute phase, rest has a very particular meaning: putting the muscles into a position of neither stretch nor contraction, and deferring any activities that require the muscle to work. If the muscle is acutely strained and very painful, this could mean a day or two in bed, either propped up on pillows in a semi-recumbent position or lying flat, whichever is most comfortable.

However, and this is an important caveat—a muscle placed at rest will atrophy, perhaps by as much as 10 percent with a single day of complete rest. This can lead to a disastrous state of profound weakness if resting is continued past the amount necessary. So resting a muscle may be a necessary strategy when the muscle is suddenly injured, but cannot be a successful strategy for long-term management of pain that lasts more than a few days.

First Aid for Acute Muscle Strain

Rest

Ice

Compression

Elevation

Medication

Avoid These Household Tasks During Recovery

- Vacuuming
- Mopping
- Cleaning bathtubs
- Shoveling (snow, dirt)

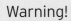

Warning!

Reprogramming May be Necessary Unhealthy patterns of back use are strongly associated with persistent back pain. For most people, back muscle injury is caused by a combination of back-stressing activities together with inactivity in the first place. Learning how to have a healthy back is important for preventing re-injury. Such activity reprogramming is usually best directed by a qualified physical therapist.

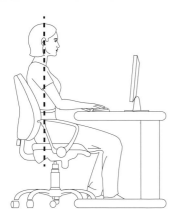

▲ Proper posture at a computer. Sit upright or slightly back directly in front of your workstation to reduce back muscle strain.

How to resolve the problem of chronic muscle strain? P-O-S-T-U-R-E. Sorry to say it, but positioning and ergonomics (see Chapter 16) play a major role in preventing chronic back strain and injury. Sitting with the back supported, the feet squarely on the ground, and trunk facing forward is fundamentally important for reducing chronic muscle strain. Likewise, proper lifting technique, re-learning how to rise from a bed, and re-engineering how you accomplish many tasks of daily living will contribute to your long term success in avoiding acute and chronic back muscle strain.

Resting for back pain got a bad reputation because years ago patients were put to bed rest for prolonged periods of time after a back injury. It turned out that prolonged bed rest was not very helpful for back pain and could in fact worsen the likelihood of chronic disability. Unfortunately, the pendulum has now swung very far in the opposite direction; many doctors have been trained to utterly reject rest as a therapeutic modality. This is not correct either, as rest has a place in the treatment of certain types of back pain. The real challenge is recognizing when and where back rest is appropriate.

In the case of muscle strain, the period of rest varies with the severity of the injury. In most cases, two to three days of rest is all that is needed. This is not to say that with severe muscle strain, longer periods of rest aren't needed. A severely strained or torn muscle will take weeks to recover. Most of the time, severe muscle strain occurs when there is a clear precipitant such as a previous injury, the kinds of strains that are seen in competitive athletic settings. If you have not been training for a triathlon or engaged in vigorous athletics and you find that your back still hurts after two or three days of resting what you think is a muscle strain, you should seek a medical opinion.

ICE IS MORE THAN NICE

Ice is the best friend we have for acute injury. In the case of managing back pain, ice is a two-for-one special: it controls inflammation and blocks pain signaling. When using ice, it's best to limit any one treatment period to 20 minutes; this will reduce the potential for damage to the skin and soft tissues. When back muscle strain first happens, it will be necessary to ice the muscle several times in a day. Five to seven treatments of 20 minutes each are not unusual.

The sooner you can apply the ice after injury, the better. Getting ice on a muscle strain "in the field" is ideal, but ice is beneficial at any point within the first 24 to 48 hours after a muscle strain injury. Everyone should have an icy gel-pack in the freezer ready to go for occasional household bumps and bruises, but if you have back pain and muscle strain, a supply of two ice packs means that one can be in use while the other is cooling back down.

Ice can be used by many people even after the 48-hour time window has passed. The inflammatory response to an injury such as muscle strain is really set in motion during the first several hours, but is hardly complete by 48 hours. In fact, if muscle fibers are actually damaged and the immune system is activated in response, the inflammatory cells are still flooding into the damaged area at 48 hours, and will probably remain present in markedly increased numbers for a week or more. Some people find that once the first 48 hours after an injury have passed that warm compresses are more effective.

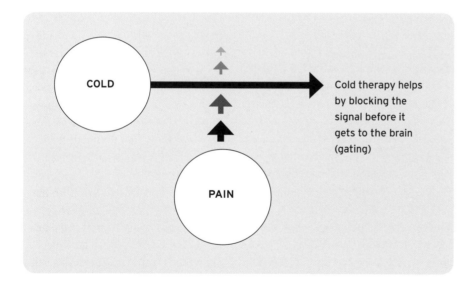

COLD

Cold therapy helps by blocking the signal before it gets to the brain (gating)

PAIN

Warning!

Insulate the Ice Ice should be applied to the body wrapped in a light cloth or dish towel. It's best to use a moldable gel pack to get the maximum contact with the body surface, but if you use ice cubes, put them in an icepack with just enough cold water so that when the icepack is on the body, the water is helping to deliver the cold from the ice.

It is important to note that if the ice is too cold, the cold of the ice will itself be painful and possibly cause harm. The solution for this is to wrap another layer of light cloth around the icepack; t-shirts and dishtowels are great for this purpose. A lightly wrapped icepack can be inconspicuously tucked into a waistband. There are even icepacks that strap to the back of a chair with elastic bands. Car trips are notorious for exacerbating back pain; next time you take a trip, take along an icepack and see if that doesn't help.

Drug-Free Painkiller

Many of my patients are initially skeptical about the benefits of ice. However, for muscle and joint-related pain, ice is a safe, effective treatment that relieves pain and reduces inflammation. How does ice relieve pain? Acutely, the ice (when wrapped in a light cloth) cools the skin to the point of activating the "cool-cold" receptors. These cool-cold receptors are located on nerves that send signals fairly rapidly to the spinal cord. When the cool-cold signals reach the spinal cord, they essentially close the gate on the slower-traveling pain signals. Thus, the cooling of a body area makes it more difficult for pain signals to penetrate into the spinal cord, where they would gain access to the pathways leading to the brain and our conscious awareness of pain.

COMPRESSION CAN HELP

The *C* in RICE-M stands for compression. Compression helps reduce the amount of swelling that occurs after an injury such as a strain. In addition, compression helps to immobilize the injured structure and allow the repair process to take place without additional injury incurred by excessive movement.

Swelling is a normal consequence of injury, part of the inflammatory response. Swelling occurs in part because some of the injury response signals lead the neighboring blood vessels to become leaky, almost like a soaker hose in the garden. The fluid component of blood can then exit the vessels (plasma extravasation) and enter the surrounding tissues. Swelling is potentially helpful because it can lead to a state of relative immobilization. For example, think how hard it can be to bend a finger that's been swollen by a bee-sting. But while immobilization is generally valuable after some injuries, the swelling is often painful. Thus, preventing excessive swelling is sometimes a critical component of controlling pain. Excessive swelling can also impede the blood supply to the area and may disrupt the normal architecture of the injured tissues. For back muscles, compression can be applied with a folded over towel pressed up against the painful part.

ELEVATION IN BACK MUSCLE INJURY

The *E* in RICE-M is for elevation. It sounds silly, doesn't it, to picture someone trying to elevate their back after a muscle strain injury. In fact, if you can't elevate your injured back muscle without stretching, don't try. For the first few days, the back needs to rest, and stretching it would be counter to that primary need. Perhaps the best you can accomplish is to avoid putting the injured part lower than the rest of the body for the first period after the muscle strain.

The best way for most people to rest the spine is to lie with their backs on the floor and the legs propped up on a chair or sofa with the knees bent at 90 degrees. When you have acutely strained a specific back muscle, lying may not be the best position. It may be necessary to adopt a side-lying position, with the hips and knees bent to reduce tension on the spine. Your best bet may be side-lying on the uninjured side. Remember that with side-lying, many people find it necessary to place a pillow between the knees to reduce excess tension on the hips. With side-lying, you can put the injured side up so it is elevated more than half of the body. If your back is otherwise healthy, it may be possible for you to comfortably lie on your stomach, perhaps with a pillow or two under your abdomen for support. In this case, go right ahead and lie on the stomach with the back fully elevated.

MEDICATIONS SPEED RECOVERY

The big *M* in RICE-M is for medication. In the context of muscle strain, the medications of choice are the nonsteroidal anti-inflammatory drugs, or NSAIDs. You have probably taken NSAIDs before. The most commonly available is ibuprofen, which is marketed under the trade names Advil and Motrin. Ibuprofen is one of a class of medications that not only interfere with pain signaling but also interrupt the inflammatory cascade that follows an injury. Other medications in the NSAID family available over the counter include naproxen, sold as Aleve or Naprosyn. There are also stronger NSAIDs available by prescription, including higher strength tablets of ibuprofen.

Other medications against pain are generally lacking in anti-inflammatory benefits. Acetaminophen, for example, is quite effective against mild-to-moderate pain, but doesn't provide the anti-inflammatory benefits of NSAIDs. There is some evidence to suggest that in some settings, morphine, the primary opioid, is actually pro-inflammatory, which should not discourage its appropriate use, but means it would not be effective in reducing inflammation, one of the goals of early treatment for muscle strain.

MULTIMODAL TREATMENT WORKS BEST

The limitations of NSAIDs are partly why it is so important to implement a comprehensive treatment strategy using all the parts of the RICE-M approach and not just take some pills and soldier on. It seems obvious but, if you think that pills will solve all your problems, you will probably wind up in more trouble than you imagined possible. That said, if you have a muscle strain and if your doctor or back care specialist says it's okay for you to take NSAIDs, then these can be an essential part of your response to back muscle strain. You may need to take them every day for the first few days after injury, but if you take NSAIDs for more than three days, you should discuss it with a healthcare provider to make sure that risks and benefits are being properly balanced.

Phase 2: Exercises for Restoring and Strengthening the Back

There is no one best exercise for your back.[3] Two types of exercise are essential when you want to increase your back's resistance to injury: those that strengthen the abdominals and others that strengthen the intrinsic back muscles. The best exercises are abdominal crunches and, for lack of a better term, back crunches.

Warning!

GI Side Effects The tremendous usefulness of NSAIDs is limited by their side effects, the most troubling of which is the heavy toll these medicines have on the stomach and GI tract. All of the NSAIDs increase the chances of developing gastric bleeding; statistics suggest that perhaps 30,000 people a year have serious health problems as a result of GI bleeding after taking NSAIDs. These medications can also be hard on the kidneys, and chronic use for more than a short period should be implemented on the advice of a physician with sound knowledge of how to minimize the risks (taking the medication with some food) and how to monitor for signs of trouble (blood or other changes in the bowel movements, increases in blood pressure).

What's New: Back to Basic Pain Meds

Troubling setbacks have followed new discoveries in more selective anti-inflammatory drugs. Referred to as the COX-2 inhibitors because of their ability to more selectively inhibit Cyclooxygenase-2 (as opposed to inhibiting both COX-1 and COX-2), these drugs were highly effective for many people with chronic inflammatory pain conditions such as osteoarthritis and degenerative joint disease. For some, the effects of these medications were nothing short of miraculous, restoring levels of function and activity that had seemed permanently beyond reach. There was even evidence to suggest that people might do better after surgery if these medicines were given just beforehand.

Unfortunately, at least some the medicines in this group increased the risk of heart attack, a risk that no one was willing to accept. After many deaths, a huge public outcry, and untold sums of money spent, some of these medicines have been withdrawn from the market and the use of others, including Celebrex, has become much more limited in scope. The bottom line is that for most people, a moderate dose of ibuprofen taken with food is a generally safe and effective choice for treating back muscle strain.

The ability to do these exercises is determined by your overall back health. If you have recently had a back injury, whether from an accident or another more minor incident, being able to do abdominal crunches and back crunches may be a long-term treatment goal rather than a currently realistic expectation. Check with your physical therapist about how to adapt these exercises to your limitations.

ABDOMINAL CRUNCHES

Abdominal crunches are a beautiful thing, as mundane as they sometimes seem. The health benefits of this exercise are multiple and essential for a happy life: abdominal crunches will not only strengthen your back but will also improve posture and trim the waistline. Improved posture will greatly enhance your resistance to back injury, and a trim waistline has been associated with reduced likelihood of serious heart disease! Once your back is on the mend from any acute problems, abdominal crunches should be a part of your daily routine. My dad, a lifelong health and fitness aficionado and mentor, has been known to do 400 abdominal crunches a day, three times a week. I usually scrape by with around 30 a day, and even a few is better than none.

In the simplest form, the abdominal crunch consists of lying on the back with the hips and knees bent. The feet should be flat on the floor. Holding the pelvis in neutral position, the abdominal muscles are gradually tightened bringing the head up and the shoulders up off the floor. The muscles are then relaxed gradually and the head and shoulders lowered back to the floor. The middle of the back should not rise up far from the floor, as doing a full sit-up is really taxing on the lower back.

There are some differences of opinion about what to do with the arms in abdominal crunches. Some people leave the arms at the side, while others cross them across the chest, and others place the hands behind the head. It is really a matter of personal preference, and the most important point is to minimize whatever barriers might exist for someone doing this exercise. If you prefer the hands at the sides, then by all means, keep them there. If you want to cross your arms across your chest, this probably adds to the challenge. If you do chose to place the hands behind the head, take care not to apply pressure to the head, as this will strain the neck. Never use the hands to pull the head forward.

Once you have a routine of performing several abdominal crunches at least three times a week, you can begin to try some variations by doing oblique crunches or by starting from a flat position and bringing the legs up together with the head and shoulders. You can even do oblique crunches with the bent elbows reaching across to meet the opposite knee, but that's getting really fancy. If your back has been injured, you will probably have to start with a basic pelvic tilt series and build up to the basic abdominal crunch. You may find that a mat or padded surface is necessary for you to be comfortable doing crunches. The most essential point is for you to do whatever it takes to get the basic abdominal crunches into your everyday routine.

BACK CRUNCHES

Before Pilates, many healthy people were not paying enough attention to their core muscles. Now, there are lots of really cool exercises you can do to strengthen your core and increase your resistance to back muscle strain. Many of these are highlighted in Chapter 14. If you ask me which exercise would I recommend, it would be what is known in Yoga as the modified locust. In the midwest, this might be called the "Mayo exercise." Lying on your abdomen, place a pillow under your stomach, so that you can lie comfortably. Stretch your arms out on the floor extending past your head and point your toes so that your legs are flat on the floor also. Contracting the back muscles, raise your arms and legs off the floor at the same time, and raise your head up as well. Hold this position for a several seconds and then relax gradually back down to the floor. Repeat this exercise several times, gradually increasing the amount of time that you hold the back crunch.

Many adaptations of the back crunch have been developed to recondition the back after an injury. If you are recovering from an acute episode of back pain, talk about this with your doctor or physical therapist and obtain their guidance on how you can progress toward improved strength in the back extensor muscles. Some variations of the exercise include raising one arm and the opposite leg, while others progress by first raising the upper body with the support of the arms. The back crunch is a beautiful and profoundly empowering exercise to do; it should be a part of those things you do just for yourself every day. Strengthening the back extensors is an essential part of increasing your back's resistance to muscle strain and other injury.

 Warning!

Recover Fully Before Doing Back Crunches Doing the back crunch is only possible once you have fully recovered from a back injury and it is not to be performed during the first week after an acute back muscle strain. The acutely strained back muscle should be rested, and this exercise is not compatible with muscle resting.

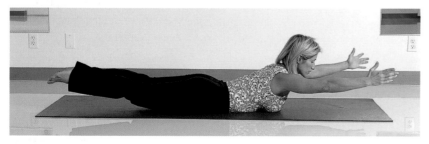

▲ A back crunch

Phase 3: Six Steps to Prevent Chronic Back Muscle Strain

1. USE PROPER POSTURE

Proper posture is vitally important when sitting and when lifting. You will read later in this chapter about the consequences of sustaining a flexed spine position for more than a couple of minutes: ligament fatigue leading to muscle spasm leading to pain and more maladaptive postures. Sitting, standing, and bending with proper posture are essential for staying free from back muscle problems. (See Chapter 16 on Ergonomics to learn more about optimizing your back health.)

2. AVOID TWISTING MOTIONS AND PAY ATTENTION TO SYMMETRY

One of the functions of the back is to support the upper body. This means that even when you are not doing any lifting, the back is carrying a load of several dozen pounds. For this reason, twisting in a funny way can place excessive strain on some of the smaller back muscles. If you have to do a task routinely or for many hours, think about how you carry out that task and try to adapt the task to your body's position. If you are loading groceries, think about how you are twisting and turning. If you are working at a computer keyboard, focus on sitting straight forward; arrange your workspace that you're not twisting to reach the keyboard or turning the head to see the computer screen fully.

3. STRETCH ROUTINELY

As emphasized in this chapter and throughout the book, stretching is essential to maintaining back health. For the muscles, stretching must be a vital part of every day's routine. Muscles that are used or required to stay in a contracted state for prolonged periods eventually shorten to accommodate that position. When you change position, those muscles may not stretch sufficiently to accommodate proper spinal alignment in the new position. Stretching daily will allow the muscles to work cooperatively and will reduce strain on other structures such as discs and joints in the back. For most people, hamstring, calf, and iliopsoas (inner hip) muscles must be stretched several times a week to maintain a proper state of flexibility and a stable standing posture.

4. LOSE POUNDS IF YOU'RE OVERWEIGHT

Carrying excess weight is a strain on the back that never goes away. For someone who is overweight, every step places additional stress on the muscles and other back structures. If you are overweight, getting your life back on track must include changing your diet to reduce your weight. There are many unproven approaches to losing weight but the universal truth is that weight loss most consistently occurs when intake is reduced and activity is increased. Increasing aerobic activity may be very difficult when you are experiencing acute back pain. Make sure to eliminate the junk foods that don't contribute to you getting vital nutrients and fiber. Increasing your consumption of fresh vegetables is usually a great first step. Fresh fruits are important too, but some people will load up on fresh fruit to the exclusion of other parts of their diet, and this is not a successful weight-loss strategy.

5. CHANGE POSITION FREQUENTLY

If you're sitting for several hours to do a task, you should get up for 10 minutes of every hour. But even as you are sitting for the other 50 minutes, make sure you are shifting from time to time, stretching a little in place and giving the muscles a little inspiration. If you are standing for long periods, make sure to shift your weight from side to side, lean against a wall for a little bit or do some quad stretches in place. The message here is that muscles need to move at least a little to avoid progressive stiffness, and in the worst case, atrophy.

6. LEARN ABOUT TRIGGER POINTS AND TRY SOME ACUPRESSURE

The back muscles are prone to muscle spasms. Trigger point approaches can by very useful for understanding why certain parts of the back have the most pain. Sometimes the answers are surprising. Learning about trigger points will help you identify certain muscles of the back and how these muscles respond to strain, stress, and pain. You can then use this knowledge to massage the trigger point that a muscle is responding with. Even if that muscle is not the root cause of the problem, reducing muscle trigger points will help control the overall pain burden that you or someone you love is experiencing with back pain. To learn more about trigger points, read on!

The Three S's of Back Muscle Health

Stretching – needed to maintain flexibility

Strengthening – all else depends on this

Symmetry – the key to staying pain-free

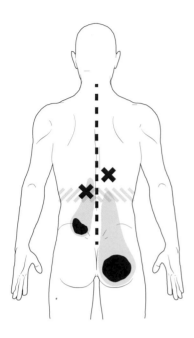

▲ Trigger points (such as these, marked with an X) result in pain that is most intense some distance away (marked with shading). [5]

Trigger Points

- Are usually painful, especially when firm pressure is applied

- Are typically palpable as areas of increased firmness in muscle

- May respond to therapeutic massage or other treatments

What Are Trigger Points?

Trigger points are shrouded in some controversy. In past years, trigger points were poorly accepted by skeptical clinicians and researchers. At the same time, they have been widely recognized by those who perform massage and manual therapies, and the pendulum is swinging toward a wider acknowledgement of trigger points as an important abnormality in muscle function. To some degree, the trigger point has eluded laboratory study because muscle is dynamic, and trigger points especially so.

Nonetheless, trigger points were characterized in detail by Janet Travell and David Simons.[4] Travell served as the White House physician during the Kennedy administration and over the course of several decades, made seminal contributions to the clinical science of musculoskeletal pain. Simons, originally an aerospace physician, brought scientific rigor to the study of trigger points, working closely with Travell in the writing of the their highly influential medical text on trigger points. Recent studies from the NIH have added scientific support for the presence of pro-inflammatory molecules and enhanced pain signals in active trigger points. In short, the trigger point is a place in the muscle that is holding an abnormally sustained contraction. This part of the muscle becomes painful to targeted pressure and sometimes is palpable as a firm area within the more pliable mass of the surrounding muscle.

HOW ARE TRIGGER POINTS TREATED?

Trigger points treated with a series of therapeutic interventions that range from acupressure massage techniques to controlled stretching to injections with local anesthetics or saline. The approach to trigger point therapy will depend on the experience and inclinations of the clinical specialist you are seeing. Although trigger points can be successfully treated by highly motivated patients themselves by applying focused pressure on the muscle, physical therapists often use a combination of approaches including trigger point massage, electrical stimulation of muscle, and "spray and stretch" techniques. In the "spray and stretch" approach, a cooling spray is applied to the skin overlying a particular trigger point, and then the muscle is rapidly stretched in a controlled manner. Trigger point injections are usually performed by certified pain specialists or others with special training in this methodology. They can provide rapid relief of pain associated with this process.

There are several books available for learning more about trigger points. One exceptional book is the *Trigger Point Therapy Workbook* by Clair Davies.[6] The author tells the amazing story of how his career as a piano tuner prepared him for his subsequent work in manual therapy. It seems that his experience of working out the relationships between the stretched wires of the piano made him very receptive to developing a detailed awareness of muscle fibers in relation to one another. His book guides the reader through the process of learning acupressure massage and gives detailed instructions for treating a wide variety of trigger point-related pains.

Trigger Point Therapies:

- Acupressure massage
- "Spray and stretch"
- Electrical stimulation
- Injections
- "Dry needling"

Testing for Back Muscle Pain

When a back problem is due to back muscle injury, most of the time the evaluation will not require expensive diagnostic tests. An experienced practitioner will be able to detect signs of muscle injury just by examining someone physically. Although severe muscle injury may be detectable using an MRI, especially when a sprain or ligamentous injury has also occurred, this mode of testing is rarely required to establish a muscle injury diagnosis. Electrical testing of a muscle and nerve would only be required if another cause of back pain was also suspected.

The Explanation

Back muscle injury, also called *back strain*, is the most common cause of temporary back pain. Although often minimized by those who never experienced it, the pain of muscle strain can be surprisingly severe and may disable a person from doing even basic tasks for a period of days to weeks.

WHY DOES BACK MUSCLE INJURY HAPPEN?

The muscles of the back are central to the stability and strength of the back. All too often, we ask our muscles to work for us, but never "pay them back." When a person starts to cut corners and doesn't invest appropriate time and energy into staying strong and healthy, acute or chronic injury to the muscles, tendons, and ligaments often produces disabling pain and weakness. Research indicates that periods of increased demand on back muscles must be balanced with periods of rest to avoid muscle strain and chronic muscle spasms. To reach a higher level of back fitness and function, make sure that you are balancing the demands on your back with healthy opportunities for growth and play.

MUSCLES OF THE BACK

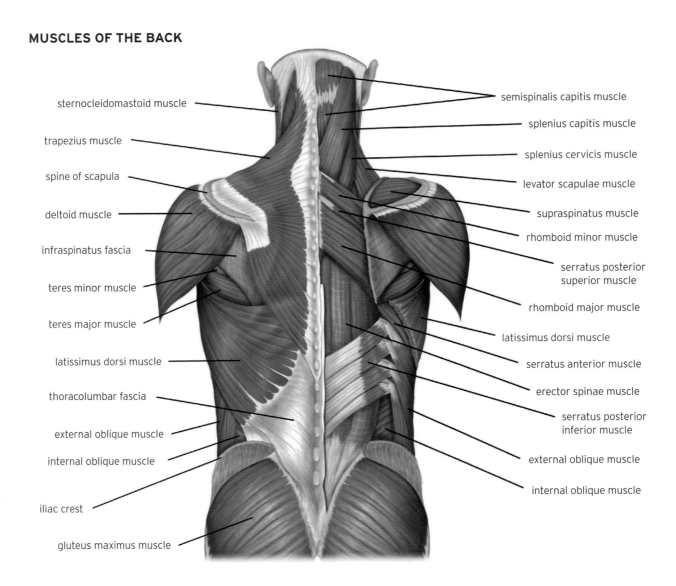

sternocleidomastoid muscle

trapezius muscle

spine of scapula

deltoid muscle

infraspinatus fascia

teres minor muscle

teres major muscle

latissimus dorsi muscle

thoracolumbar fascia

external oblique muscle

internal oblique muscle

iliac crest

gluteus maximus muscle

semispinalis capitis muscle

splenius capitis muscle

splenius cervicis muscle

levator scapulae muscle

supraspinatus muscle

rhomboid minor muscle

serratus posterior
superior muscle

rhomboid major muscle

latissimus dorsi muscle

serratus anterior muscle

erector spinae muscle

serratus posterior
inferior muscle

external oblique muscle

internal oblique muscle

If you watch young children at play, they are constantly running, jumping, bending, climbing, and crawling! These natural activities all test and challenge the back, but also build strength and resilience. For better or worse, our society places a premium on highly structured activities for adults, and we rarely get the chance to move about spontaneously and with unforced vigor. Many of us work at jobs that don't allow us to move about freely; we either have to repeat the same tasks over and over, sit at our desks for hours upon hours, or lift heavy objects without adequate assistance or training. All of these activities leave us prone to back strain.

SPRAINS AND STRAINS

A strain is an injury to a muscle (or tendon), whereas a sprain is an injury to a ligament. Tendons and ligaments are both fibrous but serve different functions. Tendons are involved in connecting muscles to bones. They have poor blood supply but are capable of feeling pain when injured or inflamed. The pain of tendonitis can be quite severe and disabling. Tendonitis often arises in people who are performing strength-requiring tasks repeatedly. Although the classic example of tendonitis is tennis elbow, more mundane tasks such as assisting with wheelchair transfers can produce this syndrome. Although more common sites for tendonitis include the elbow and knee, it is possible to have tendonitis in the back and shoulder muscles.

Ligaments are involved in connecting bone to bone. There are many important ligaments in the back, including those that hold the vertebrae to one another. These ligaments can be damaged by sharp blows, very sudden stretching movements, penetrating wounds, or other traumas. Ligaments are slow to repair and can require prolonged casting or immobilization to heal properly. Because ligaments play a fundamental role in stabilizing bones and preventing excessive movement in associated structures, chronic pain can result when damage to ligaments goes unrepaired. Instability of the spinal column has a profound impact on back function and back pain; for more information about this, see Chapter 6.

Causes of Acute Muscle Strain

- Sports injury
- Lifting
- Twisting
- Any sudden stretch

Muscle Strain Leads to:

- Weakness (lasting for days to a week)
- Pain
- Inflammation
- Persistent damage when severe
- Adaptive or maladaptive postures

27

Recent research has shed important light on the connections between strain, sprain, and back pain. Muscle strain can be produced by a sudden loading force or a strong stretching of muscle. Commonly, acute muscle strain is associated with particular sports such as soccer and hockey, but ordinary lifting can be problematic for people who might be out of shape and not using proper lifting technique. The consequences of strain can be very serious for muscle, resulting in profound muscle damage, invasion of inflammatory cells, and ultimately the replacement of healthy muscle cells by collagen.

Strain of a muscle is typically very painful and always produces a loss of muscle strength. Muscle strength drops within minutes of the strain itself but typically worsens over the first 24 hours. Laboratory studies of strain suggest that muscles can produce only half of their normal power on the first day after a strain injury. Muscle power gradually returns to normal, but this can take a week or more depending on the severity of the injury.

What happens when the stresses are more chronic? The effects of staying bent over for even a few minutes can be quite serious. Although not technically producing ligamentous sprain, the consequences of improper poster and positioning are damaging to ligaments. With sustained improper spine flexion, the normally resilient ligaments of the spine stretch but don't bounce back. The technical term for this is *viscoelastic creep*, but it is reasonable to think of this as *ligament fatigue*.[7] When ligaments fatigue, the associated muscles are recruited to respond, initially attempting to support the movement. The muscles ultimately develop a predictable pattern of spasms: random bursting muscle contractions that can be detected with electromyography. Muscle spasms are typically painful, and interfere with normal movement. The spasms resulting from sustained spine flexion occur in the multifidus, spinalis, and longissimus muscles for several hours after the improper spine movement. Some research suggests that women are especially prone to the effects of ligament fatigue.

The take-home message is that fatiguing ligaments through improper posture and poor spine ergonomics results in muscle strain, inflammation, pain, and muscle spasms that last for hours and hours. Permanent damage can occur, so the importance of maintaining proper posture and never over-reaching personal strength limits is critical. Given that it can take several days to a couple weeks for the body to repair these injuries to muscles and ligaments, it's no wonder that millions of people have aching backs that never fully recover!

CRAMPS ARE DIFFERENT FROM MUSCLE SPASMS

Cramps in muscle are swiftly-evolving, unplanned contractions of the muscle. These involuntary muscle contractions are typically painful, but can often be resolved by slowly stretching the muscle. It is usually possible to feel that the muscle is hardened in the area of a cramp. Muscle cramps are more likely in the setting of various conditions such as pregnancy, low calcium, low magnesium, hypothyroidism, and dehydration. They can reflect muscle fatigue and occur after heavy exercise. The most common sites for muscle cramps are not in the back but rather in the calves (gastrocnemius), the feet muscles, the thigh (hamstrings or quadriceps), and the rib cage area, where they are responsible to the pain of having "a stitch."

The most common remedies are stretching the muscle, intentionally contracting the muscle, massage, and warm compresses. Although the precise mechanisms of cramps remain somewhat controversial, one popular theory is that cramps represent over-activity of the nerves controlling the muscle contractions. In this way, stretching the muscle or contracting the counter-acting muscles will interrupt the nerve signal to muscle and may bring the cramp to an end.

Muscle spasms are random, bursting, and sometimes sustained contractions of muscle that are typically associated with pain and decreased motion. When severe, muscle spasms can result in muscle injury, especially if sudden or forceful movements are made while the muscle is in spasm. Although there is some controversy about whether muscle spasms are palpable, it is the experience of most trained observers that muscle spasms are readily appreciated either through direct palpation or through examining for limitations in normal movements (decreased range of motion). Muscle spasms may not respond to stretching as cramps do; treatments such as ice, warmth, and pain-relievers can help. Not infrequently the treatment of muscle spasms is addressed by doctors using prescription medications. As a testament to this, muscle relaxants continue to be among the most widely prescribed medicines. The problem with muscle relaxants is that they often interfere with thinking and levels of alertness. Some of these medications are liable to abuse, and even without abuse these medications can lead to physical or psychological dependence. Use them when needed but no more often than necessary.

Where Cramps Most Often Occur

Calf muscles (charley horse)

Foot muscles

Thigh muscles

Rib muscles (stitch)

CHAPTER RESOURCES

1. Henschke, N. and C. Maher. 2006. Red flags need more evaluation. *Rheumatology* 45 (7): 920–921.

2. Bratton, R.L. 1999. Assessment and management of acute low back pain. *American Family Physician* 60 (8): 2299-308.

3. Selby, Anna. *Banish Back Pain the Pilates Way*. Thorsons, 2003.

4. Simons, David G., Janet G. Travell, and Lois S. Simons. *Travell and Simons's Myofascial Pain and Dysfunction: The Trigger Point Manual.* 2nd ed. Baltimore, MD: Williams & Wilkins, 1999.

5. Niel-Asher, Simeon. *The Concise Book of Trigger Points, Revised Edition*. Berkeley, CA: North Atlantic Books, 2008.

6. Davies, Clair. *The Trigger Point Therapy Workbook*. Oakland, CA: New Harbinger Publications, Inc., 2001.

7. Solomonow, M. 2004. Ligaments: A source of work-related musculoskeletal disorders. *Journal of Electromyography and Kinesiology* 14:49-60.

What are fasciculations?

These perceptible contractions of muscle, when wide-spread, can be a sign of serious disease such as neurological degeneration or, quite rarely, toxic poisoning. More commonly, fasciculations are part of the muscles' normal response to fatigue or result from a decline in exercise-imposed demands. Caffeine is a potent stimulus for muscle contraction and is widely used in laboratory studies of muscle activity. Sometimes it is worth investigating whether caffeine consumption is related to bothersome fasciculations. If you have new fasciculations that persist and don't seem to be related to fatigue or muscle disuse, you should discuss this with your doctor.

How does prolonged sitting affect back muscles?

One of the consequences of prolonged sitting is a tightening or mild contracture of the hip flexor muscles. This can affect the back negatively through at least two mechanisms—one through referred pain arising from the muscle itself, the other as a consequence of the negative postural adjustments that occur when these muscles are not properly flexible. This is almost an occupational hazard of the "sedentary" but mentally engaged professions such as accounting, writing, and computer programming. Because these careers require prolonged periods of sustained mental effort, often with a computer interface, the tendency is to become lost in thought and disregard the body's need to shift and move around. Sitting can also result in back muscle atrophy and chronic muscle overuse. Proper posture and ergonomic seating arrangements are critical. There are other deleterious effects of prolonged sitting for the back, especially on the vertebral discs.

How long should I wait before going to the doctor?

The amount of time you wait before seeking acute care depends on many factors, but most of all, on the intensity of pain you are experiencing and the response of that pain to the at-home therapies discussed in this chapter. If your pain is interfering with sleep or work and is not responding to the at-home therapies, then you need an appointment with your healthcare provider. If your pain is unbearable and you cannot control it enough to wait for an appointment, then you need immediate care. Your local emergency room or urgent care facility should be able to assess your pain and provide some treatments that will provide at least short-term relief.

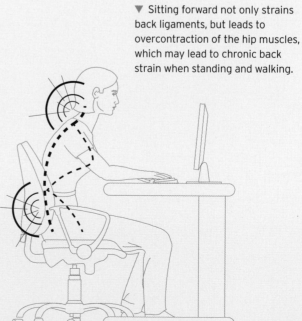

▼ Sitting forward not only strains back ligaments, but leads to overcontraction of the hip muscles, which may lead to chronic back strain when standing and walking.

CHAPTER 2

Disc Herniation

(Slipped Disc)

Seek out expert medical care and get proper diagnostic tests such as an MRI or nerve conduction test.

the DIAGNOSIS

> **Do you have pain that is located to one side of the spine?**

> **Does your pain seem to shoot down the leg, radiate into the groin or wrap around the body?**

What's New: A Changing Definition

Traditional descriptions of radiating back pain emphasize that it is more likely to be due to a compressed nerve root (and disc herniation) when the pain going into the leg extends below the knee. Recent studies indicate that even if the pain just extends into the thigh, pain could still be due to nerve root compression. [1]

Pain that radiates into the leg or groin is usually due to a nerve injury, often from a herniated disc. Back pain is called *radiating* when there is an element of pain in the back and in the leg. The degree of pain in the back due to a herniated disc is often described as rather minor; however, pain may be prominent and centrally located in the back if a disc has been previously damaged. Some people with radiating back pain have the sensation that the back and leg pains are physically connected to each other, while others have back pain and leg pains that are felt at the same time without a physical bridge of pain connecting them (there and there but not in between).

Sometimes, certain movements will make the pain worse. One way to test for a nerve root injury is to do the following (you will need a helper to do this test): sit down in a hard chair that has a straight back. The chair height should be such that your feet are firmly on the ground with your knees at a 90-degree angle. Have your helper gently take one ankle and pull it slowly outward and up. If your back pain suddenly increases with this movement, stop immediately. You may have nerve root compression; read on!

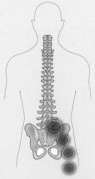

33

the PRESCRIPTION

The Good News

- People with herniated discs often do better than those with other back problems.

- Surgery can be very effective at restoring people with herniated discs to full health.

Back pain due to a pinched nerve needs expert medical assessment and care. Many times, an MRI of the back or even a CT scan will be needed as a first diagnostic test. Some doctors still prefer to start with an X-ray, but this will only show the bones and does not indicate what is happening with the disc. If your doctor recommends an MRI and you suffer from claustrophobia, make sure to let your doctor know. For most people, Magnetic Resonance Imaging is very safe.

Your doctor may also order a nerve conduction test to evaluate the integrity of the nerves arising from the spine. This test and MRIs are discussed in detail later in this chapter. Once imaging and electrical test results are in, a clearer picture will emerge. The possibilities range from "nothing is wrong" to a "slipped disc" to a "broken back."

If you have a herniated disc (sometimes referred to as a *slipped disc*):

- Your doctor may recommend physical therapy, especially if there is no perceptible weakness. Surgery may be needed if non-surgical treatments are not effective after a fair trial.
- Your doctor may refer you to a surgeon, especially if there is weakness due to nerve damage. Surgery has pluses and minuses, but in cases of weakness or incontinence, surgery may be needed urgently to preserve function.

For an isolated disc herniation, microsurgery may be the answer.

- Microsurgery is surgery through one or more small incisions.
- Recovery times are usually faster.

For many reasons, microsurgery may not be an option.

- Routine surgery for herniated discs is very effective.
- Make sure to ask about expected recovery times.
- When damage to the spine is more extensive, a more involved surgery is needed that may involve fusing adjacent spinal bones with metal hardware or bone.

AREA OF INJURY

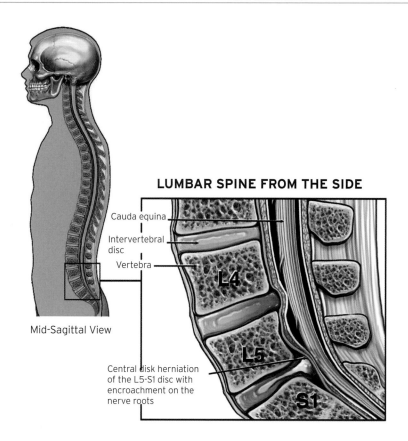

Mid-Sagittal View

LUMBAR SPINE FROM THE SIDE

Cauda equina

Intervertebral disc

Vertebra

L4

L5

S1

Central disk herniation of the L5-S1 disc with encroachment on the nerve roots

WHAT IF YOUR DOCTOR DIAGNOSES A BULGING DISC?

In this case, physical therapy and exercise are usually best. The degree of pain and disability associated with type of injury varies greatly, but in this case you can do a lot to improve your chances of a fast and full recovery. (See Chapter 5 to learn how to manage a bulging disc.)

WHAT IF YOUR DOCTOR FINDS A NERVE ROOT BEING COMPRESSED BY AN OVERGROWTH OF BONES (BONY SPURS) OR LIGAMENTS IN THE LOWER BACK?

The overgrowth of bones and ligaments in the lower back is usually the end result of years of accumulated trauma to the back, and carries the label of degenerative joint disease (DJD). Surgery may be an option, but this depends on the extent of damage to the spine. Many times, physical therapy and programmed exercise is the right solution.

Rare Causes of Root Compression

In rare cases, nerve root compression is due to a mass (tumor), an infection (abcess), or a spinal malformation. These causes of nerve root compression are readily assessed through MRI and the other diagnostic tests described here. The treatment for these conditions is individualized.

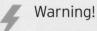

Warning!

Don't Wait Weeks for Help
Unfortunately, many doctors have been trained to wait six weeks before pursuing a fuller work up with MRI or EMG tests for a suspected disc herniation. The pain of disc herniation is usually severe enough that six weeks is far too long for anyone to remain in agony. So if you are in a lot of pain, and especially if you have weakness as well, don't accept treatment that you think is second rate. Tell your provider you need a proper work up or go elsewhere for help.[2]

The Treatment

If your doctor recommends physical therapy first, it usually means you have the type of disc herniation that is best treated without surgery.[3] There are several treatment modalities that fall under the umbrella of physical therapy as the primary treatment for disc problems: thermal therapies, electrical stimulation therapies, manual therapies, traction/inversion therapies, conditioning, and strengthening.

THERMAL THERAPIES REDUCE PAIN

Warm compresses, cold packs or both in combination can be very effective at reducing pain levels.[4] Pain control is an important part of early treatment for disc problems. Pain levels with disc herniations can average 8 on a scale of 10 and will be higher with movement or stress. Pain can induce compensatory postures and movements that may increase disc pressures and slow progress toward recovery.

ELECTRICAL STIMULATION THERAPIES RELAX MUSCLES

Electrical stimulation may be used on selected muscle groups to induce muscle relaxation through a "fatigue" mechanism. The electrical stimulation can be applied in areas where muscle spasms are contributing to the pressures on the disc as well as on overactive muscles that are perpetuating abnormal postures.

MANUAL THERAPIES RELIEVE AND REALIGN

Proper alignment of the spine and normal postures are essential to normalizing pressures on vertebral discs. In the thoracic spine, a pinched nerve can produce muscle spasm profound enough to interfere with proper breathing. Trigger point therapy is designed to relax muscles that have abnormal zones of muscle fiber contractions known as *trigger points*. Low-velocity manipulations can adjust dislocated sacroiliac joints or misaligned facet joints. In some cases, extension of the spine may provide pain relief from pain due to disc disease.[5]

TRACTION AND INVERSION THERAPIES RELEASE PRESSURE

Releasing pressure on a disc increases the likelihood that it will return to its regular configuration.[6] For some people, inversion can be carried out successfully at home, but for most, a supervised course of traction or inversion therapy is safest. For the person determined to try inversion therapy at home, it is possible to purchase an inversion table. For milder forms of inversion, an inclined board with padding may produce some benefits. For someone with active back pain, though, getting into position on an inclined board may represent a substantial challenge.

CONDITIONING IS CORE TO BACK HEALTH

Strengthening and conditioning are essential parts of physical therapy for disc problems whether or not surgery is undertaken. I often tell patients that they should expect to work hard at getting better from a back injury. I really discourage people from taking time off from work for back problems unless they are attending physical therapy and dedicating themselves to getting better through supervised exercise. If you have a herniated disc with radiating leg pain, a physical therapist will need to guide your first steps in back strengthening. In most cases where the disc herniation is not causing actual weakness, physical therapy is the preferred treatment.

Physical therapy is highly effective for many types of back problems, including some herniated discs. There are several advantages to pursuing physical therapy, but the primary advantage is that it avoids the complications of surgery and may be completely effective.[7,8]

It is not yet clear whether physical therapy is more cost-effective or time-efficient than surgery. The usual medical perspective is that for disc herniations causing muscle weakness, back surgery is more likely to be effective than not. For disc herniations where pain is the predominating problem *and* there is no demonstrable weakness due to apparent nerve injury, surgery will be considered as a second-line option for particularly severe situations.[9]

Know When to Seek a Second Opinion

If you think you have disc-related weakness and your doctor has recommended not pursuing surgery, make sure you understand why not. Make sure the doctor has examined the muscles that you believe to be weak, and if after communicating clearly about any perceived weakness, you don't feel understood, seek a second opinion.

Sometimes severe pain can cause muscles to function poorly, and this may be difficult to distinguish from the worrisome weakness that arises from direct nerve damage. The distinction is important and critically so in patients with disc herniation. Often, an electromyographic (EMG) study of the muscles can distinguish pain-induced weakness from nerve damage-induced weakness.

TO-DO LIST FOR SURGERY

If your doctor refers you to a surgeon right away, chances are that you have a nerve root or roots that would be in danger without surgical decompression. Typically, surgery is needed if the herniated disc is pressing on a nerve and causing weakness in one or several muscles. Pain is also usually present, but the surgery that is needed to protect the function of the nerve root will typically relieve much of the pain.[10]

When you go to see the surgeon, there are several things you should do to prepare for the visit: gathering records, making a list of potential questions, and lining up a support person to go along on the visit.

First, make sure that you have copies of any X-rays, CT scans, MRIs, or myelograms with you or arrange for these to be sent directly to the surgeon's office. You will need copies of recent blood work and documentation of any other medical conditions you may have. Take a detailed list of medications that you are prescribed and include in this any dietary supplements that you take.

Second, write down a list of questions that you may have about your back problem and the planned procedure. These question lists are well known to most physicians; try to weed out the routine ones and identify the questions that are most critical to you. You can learn a lot about your back problem and the usual approaches to treatment before your appointment with the surgeon; as you do this, some of your initial questions may be answered but new ones will arise. Your surgeon may direct you to specific educational resources. Some spine practices have websites that are designed to provide routine information about treatments and surgeries. Your public library may have excellent resource materials ranging from books to videos.

A SECOND PAIR OF EARS

You will need a support person to accompany you to the surgeon's visit. Everyone who visits a specialist doctor should plan on having a "second pair of ears." In some extreme cases in which no one is available, you can take an audio recording device along. Make sure to ask the doctor if they are comfortable with a recording being made. The recording device, while useful, is not as good as a friend or a family member, who will often be able to ask important questions and provide emotional support if the news is bad.

Make sure you have a clear idea of the surgery that is planned. There are several possible surgical approaches that can be used for the treatment of a herniated disc. The extent of surgery will vary with the extent of back disease; for problems limited to a simple herniated disc, the planned surgery should be limited, but the specific approach will depend on the particular expertise of the surgeon and should be guided by his or her best judgment. The approaches used include an open discectomy, a micro-discectomy, and micro-endoscopic discectomy.

OPEN DISCECTOMY

Open discectomy is the oldest, more established procedure. It involves an incision, perhaps two to three inches in length. Through this vertical incision on the back, the surgeon will cut or separate the layers of fat, muscle, and connective tissues that overlie the spine. There is a layer of bone that covers the spinal cord that must be passed through in order to access the spine. This bone consists of the posterior portions of the spinal vertebrae that are stacked, one on top of the other, to form a protective covering over the spinal cord. In the open discectomy, it is necessary to remove part of one of these, or parts of two adjacent vertebrae, using a technique called *laminectomy* or *hemi-laminectomy*.[11] Once the bone is removed, it may be possible for the surgeon to see the spinal cord and its covering as well as the nerve root at that level. The disc herniation is usually just on the other side of the nerve root seen through the surgical incision. Removing the herniated disc material is done with specialized cutting tools once the nerve and spinal cord are protected from harm. The spinal cord may be gently held to the side using a tool called a retractor. Once the disc herniation is removed, the surgeon will begin to close the incision, often repairing the opening in the various layers by stitching with suture thread. Sutures come in various strengths and materials, and strong sutures are used in high-load areas like the back. The skin is the final layer that must be repaired to complete the surgery, and the skin incision may be repaired with sutures, staples, or other techniques. The recovery time for the open discectomy is usually longest of the three procedures, but the method offers a wide view of the problems in the spine, and may be preferred over micro-discectomy when certain conditions apply.

Questions to Ask Your Surgeon

- Are you sure I need this surgery?

- How many of these procedures have you done?

- How long will I need to be out of work?

- How much pain should I expect after surgery?

- How long will I need to take pain medicine for afterwards?

- How long will I be in the hospital following the procedure?

- How long before I can drive again?

What's New: Disc Location May Dictate the Outcome

A recent analysis of a study on surgery for the treatment of herniated discs indicated that the effectiveness of the surgery at reducing pain depended in part on the location of the disc involved. The higher up in the low back, the better the chance of a positive outcome from surgery. It seems that the L5-S1 disc repairs were associated with less pain relief and lower levels of post-surgical functioning.[12]

What's New: Young Adults Fare Well

A recent study of people ages 20 to 35 with single-level disc herniation found that most of these young adults have great results: although five out of 67 people in the study had to have a second surgery for damage to another disc in the back, none of the people who answered the doctor's survey needed constant pain medicine, and most had returned to sports activities without undue pain.[13]

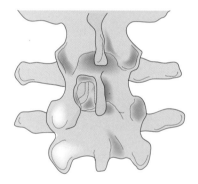

▲ The removal of bone (partial laminectomy) for a micro-discectomy

MICRO-DISCECTOMY

Like open discectomy, micro-discectomy is a procedure to remove a herniated disc but it is performed using a very small incision. Typically, a guiding catheter is positioned using an operating room X-ray machine called a fluoroscope. This guide catheter is much too small to allow the surgery to take place, so a series of progressively larger tubes are slid into place over the catheter in a process that enlarges (or dilates) the access path that the surgeon must take through the layers of fat, muscle, and connective tissue in the back. In this process, layers of fat and muscle are spread apart rather than cut, allowing for less local damage and perhaps contributing to the faster recovery times associated with this surgery. In order to visualize the disc herniation, it is still necessary to remove some of the posterior bone of the spine, so a partial laminectomy is done through the surgical access tube. A microscope is used to visualize the disc herniation as well as some of the spinal nerve elements (spinal cord and spinal nerve). The herniated disc material is removed using a specialized cutting tool that passes down through the surgical access tube. Once the disc herniation is removed, the tube can be removed with care and the incision in the skin repaired. Recovery times for micro-discectomy are generally faster than for open discectomy, although in both procedures, patients will generally begin walking the day of surgery.

MICRO-ENDOSCOPIC DISCECTOMY

▼ The procedure for a micro-endoscopic discectomy, performed through a keyhole incision

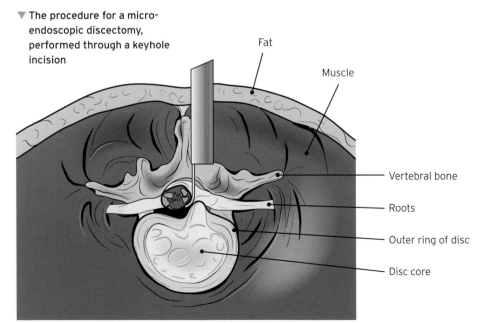

Fat

Muscle

Vertebral bone

Roots

Outer ring of disc

Disc core

Micro-endoscopic discectomy is a procedure that is similar in many respects to the micro-discectomy. Instead of positioning a microscope over the end of the tube and looking down into the incision from outside, a fiber-optic camera is passed into the tube to visualize the structures of interest. The surgical instruments need-ed to perform the removal of the disc herniation are also passed through the tube as in the micro-discectomy but must then compete for limited maneuvering space with the miniature camera.

PREPARATION FOR SURGERY

After you visit your surgeon's office for the first time, make sure to read over any materials that you receive from the doctor and the doctor's assistants or office staff. If you have any serious questions or worries, get in contact with the office and seek out advice from trusted sources. You may want to obtain a second opinion if you have lingering doubts about the plans for surgery. Once you make the decision to go forward, you will want to follow the surgeon's recommendations closely.

You will be told what to do to prepare for surgery. In most cases, you will instructed not to eat after midnight or perhaps earlier the evening before the sur-gery. Most surgeons begin operating early in the morning, so you may be checking in for the procedure before dawn. A pre-operative physical exam is often required before surgery; you may be asked to see your regular doctor for this or instructed to undergo a special pre-operative examination. Some additional tests may be or-dered at this point to make sure that the medical risks for surgery are fully known and minimized.

WHAT TO EXPECT AFTER SURGERY

The pace of recovery depends to some degree on the type of surgery that you have had for the herniated disc and on the type of work you are returning to. After an open discectomy, the time required before a return to work can be more than two weeks. The time for micro-discectomy may be sooner.

At first, it may not be possible to drive, especially after an open discectomy. Carefully follow your surgeon's instructions about driving. It stands to reason that (unless your surgeon says it's okay) no driving also means no flying airplanes, no downhill skiing, no boating, etc. It is surprising how often people with excellent common sense in other areas will try to circumvent the necessary restrictions on activity that follow back surgery. Try to remember that your back has undergone a sophisticated and expensive procedure. Your body needs time to heal and stitch itself back together; following the activity restrictions put in place by your surgeon will maximize your chances of getting a good result from surgery!

What's New: The Risks and Costs of Micro-Endoscopic Discectomy

A new study shows that micro-endoscopic discectomy may carry more risks than either open or micro-discectomy, and may in the end be more expensive.[14] Make sure that you understand the specific plan for your surgery. If you feel uncomfortable or have reservations, try to discuss these openly. A second opinion can sometimes be very helpful for making the best medical decision.

Warning! Follow Your Doctor's Orders for Limiting Activities

It is really important to respect the restrictions your surgeon places on activity following surgery. Overly aggressive "rehabilitation" outside the bounds set can cause delays in healing, a relapse of the problem, or sometimes a serious worsening in the back problem.

MEDICATIONS FOLLOWING SURGERY

Your surgeon may prescribe pain medication to control the pain after surgery. It's important to take pain medication as prescribed. Pain control is very important during the recovery period, as it will improve your chances of a good result and lessen the likelihood of persistent pain after surgery. Be sure to alert your surgeon if there is severe pain after surgery that doesn't respond to the pain medicine provided. Severe pain can be a sign of unexpected difficulties such as bleeding or infection. You will be able to gauge your need for the medications, as pain quickly escalates if a dose is skipped or delayed. For many people, the first three days after surgery are the worst from a pain perspective, and once this period passes, the need for pain medicine declines.

Most of the medications used to control post-surgical pain are in the opioid drug family. These medications are notorious for causing constipation. This constipation can be a serious problem so you'll need to have a plan in place to minimize these effects. An additional pill may be prescribed to stimulate the bowels and a stool softener may also be prescribed. Discuss measures you would normally take for constipation with your doctor, including your usual routine. Helpful steps to take might include drinking some extra water every day, taking a glass of prune juice or eating some prunes, getting some extra fiber in the diet, or taking supplements. For many people, the constipation that follows with the post-surgical pain medications won't stop until the meds themselves are no longer used.

POST-SURGICAL PHYSICAL THERAPY

Physical therapy is usually part of the recovery plan after back surgery, and a key element to making a full and successful recovery from disc herniation.It may begin with an assessment immediately after surgery, or start as late as three weeks post surgery. The inactivity that accompanied your back problem and the surgery may have weakened your back and stomach muscles. A guided program of strengthening, conditioning, and pain control is critical to preventing a relapse or recurrence of disc herniation. Ultimately, you will want to develop your own program of back exercise, but during the recovery from surgery, make sure any exercises you do are in line with the expectations of your surgeon and physical therapists.

Testing for Nerve Root Compression

The tests most commonly used to diagnose nerve root compression include the EMG/NCS and the MRI. Neither of these tests is perfect and they serve complementary purposes.

ELECTROMYOGRAPHY AND NERVE CONDUCTION STUDIES

The EMG/NCS is a fundamentally important test for determining if there is damage to the nerves or nerve roots. The EMG portion of the test involves having a slender needle placed into one or more muscles. The specially designed needle is a high performance instrument designed to measure the electrical activity of the muscle with a minimum of noise and the best possible combination of signal detection and resolution. With this needle, it is usually possible to determine if the connection between brain and muscle is working well. Sometimes it is possible to detect prior injury to a nerve. Once the needle has been placed into the muscle, the doctor may just "listen" for a short while to see whether there is spontaneous activity in the muscle. The doctor may then ask you to tighten or contract the muscle. This makes it possible to see if the muscle is responding appropriately to the signals the brain is sending. It may be necessary to reposition the needle in the same muscle, and is usually necessary to test multiple muscles in this manner.

The EMG can be instrumental for pinpointing damage to a specific nerve root. However, the test results do depend to some extent on the technique and interpretation of the person conducting the test, and sometimes the test needs to be repeated. Early after a nerve injury, the signs of injury in the muscle are not as readily apparent. This is because following a nerve injury, a series of changes take place in the muscle that the nerve supplies. These changes make it easier to detect a nerve injury but are not well established until three weeks in most cases.

Be Prepared for Pain

The EMG is painful for most people; the degree of pain varies with the person and the particular muscle being studied. The hand and biceps muscles are especially painful. It can be painful if the needle enters the muscle near the point where the nerve connects to the muscle (muscle endplate or neuromuscular junction). Although the needle does produce very minor trauma to the muscle, it is an invaluable technique for learning about how the muscles and nerve are functioning: this is something the best MRI is not capable of doing.

▼ EMG Test

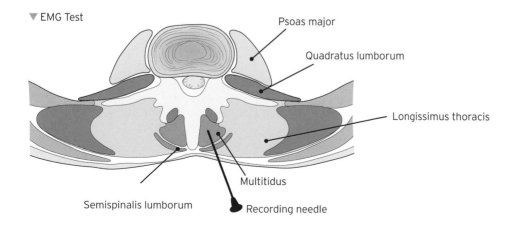

Psoas major

Quadratus lumborum

Longissimus thoracis

Multitidus

Semispinalis lumborum

Recording needle

43

If You Smoke, Stop!

If you are still smoking, now is the time to quit. Smoking will interfere with your recovery from surgery and is proven to decrease the success of surgery. Some surgeons will refuse to operate on current smokers. Smoking makes failed back syndrome (a condition where the patient has severe chronic pain even after back surgeries) more likely. Smoking will interfere with your ability to get aerobic exercise and get better from your back injury. In addition, it increases your risk for lung cancer by 10 times, increases your risk for having a heart attack, and increases health risks for those who are around you when you smoke. If you are unable to quit on your own, ask your doctor for help. One predictor of success at eventually quitting the nicotine habit is the willingness to quit again. So even if you've tried and failed before, don't be discouraged; resolve to start over.

PAINFUL BUT PURPOSEFUL NCS

The other part of the EMG/NCS series is the nerve conduction test (NCS). This test involves delivering a series of shocks to various nerves in the body and measuring the responses. The NCS usually precedes the EMG. There is currently no practical alternative to the NCS and the information obtained from the study can be invaluable for firming up a diagnosis. If your doctor suspects nerve root damage or radiculopathy, the NCS can be an important in excluding other nerve conditions and identifying specific nerve root syndromes.

For many people, the NCS is quite painful. It is often more painful for people with pre-existing nerve damage, such as that caused by diabetes. Young people are also especially susceptible to the pain of NCS, and finally, repetitive shocks are almost always much more painful than single shocks, but this depends on how closely timed the repeated shocks are. The NCS is painful because the skin not only is a barrier to the current needed to electrically stimulate the nerves underneath but it is richly innervated with pain-sensing fibers that will be directly stimulated by the electrical current.

Because the NCS can be so painful, some people have wondered if there is permanent damage. There is no evidence that NCS causes permanent damage; in fact, the NCS delivers electrical current to the nerve that activates the nerve in a very "normal" manner. In general, it has not been common practice to provide sedation or anxiety-relieving medications before the study. This may be because cooperation is required for the EMG, which is often paired with the NCS, and because some of the more common anxiety-relieving medications could interfere with some parts of the EMG study. It is best to bring a support person along to the EMG/NCS, especially if you are not someone who takes great pride in being stoic!

MAGNETIC RESONANCE IMAGING

The MRI has become an instrumental part of confirming a diagnosis of nerve root injury. In a perfect world, a classical nerve root compression syndrome would show such a consistent and specific pattern of radiating pain and focal muscle weakness arising after a simple bending injury that an MRI would not be needed. However, in the real world, there are other causes of nerve root injury that are best assessed by MRI. Herniated discs are just one of the potential causes of nerve root injury, and MRI is an excellent test for assessing for the presence of other worrisome causes of nerve root compression.

The quality of the MRI is critical for the doctors reviewing the study and making decisions about your healthcare. Make sure to check with the doctor ordering the study for any pointers to facilities with good quality MRI studies. Some centers may be using machines that are out of date or older technology that will not produce a crisp picture of your back's structures. It is also critically important to hold perfectly still during many portions of the image acquisition process, so try to listen carefully to the MRI technicians instructions once your study is underway. Ask for a copy of the study so that you can keep this and bring it with you to the relevant healthcare appointments. Make sure to request that a copy of the report be sent to you (if possible) or your primary care doctor's office, as well as to any specialist that may have requested the MRI. If you have a history of claustrophobia, this may factor into your decision to choose open over closed MRI. Early "open MRI" images were not always of the best quality because of the technological challenges involved in producing a uniform magnetic field in the open MRI configuration. The need for a strong, highly uniform magnetic field is why MRI machines tend to consist of a relatively tight fitting tube into which you slide for the study. The MRI rapidly pulses a strong magnetic field over the body and records the "relaxation" of the atomic nuclei as they reorient spontaneously when the field is very briefly switched off. This magnetization process occurs many times during the standard MRI study and accounts for the loud noise of most MRI scanners.

IS IT DANGEROUS TO HAVE AN MRI?

People often wonder if MRI is dangerous. It is not. MRI is probably the safest imaging technology available. Unlike CT scans, there is no radiation, so there is no reason to worry about MRI increasing your risk of cancer. Unlike ultrasound, there is very little energy transfer despite all the banging sounds that may emanate from the machine. The tight-fitting spaces of MRI machines and the loud noise of most scanners can be mildly intimidating and uncomfortable, but listening to music and/or maintaining a state of mental calm by focusing on the value of the test are usually sufficient to offset most worries.

Your doctor may offer premedication for the test if you express concerns, anticipate feeling claustrophobia, or have a history of anxiety with MRI. Remember that taking a pre-MRI anxiety-relieving medication probably means that you will need a driver to take you home after. Although MRI cannot "see everything," it does offer a dazzlingly detailed picture that can detect problems as small as a grain of rice. It also has the capability to detect changes in the body due to inflammation.

Warning! Make Medications Known

Because the EMG is a test that is invasive, if minimally so, it is important to make sure that the lab knows what medications you are taking in advance of the test. Especially if you are taking a blood thinner, the electrodiagnostic lab needs this information, and you should again notify the doctor before allowing the test to be done if blood-thinning medications are part of your medical regimen. If you have problems with blood clotting, it is important to make sure this part of your medical history is discussed as well.

Warning! MRI and Metals Don't Mix

If you have a pacemaker, electrical implants, or a history of working in the metals industry, you need to check with the radiology center and your doctor before having an MRI. In these situations and selected others, the presence of metal in the body can pose a hazard and means that MRI cannot be done.

WHAT HAPPENS IN THE DOCTOR'S OFFICE?

Your doctor or practitioner may perform some basic maneuvers to determine if nerve root injury is the cause of your back pain. This will probably include testing the muscles in your legs to determine if they have full strength. The practitioner may test sensation, trying to determine if there is any pattern of sensory loss. Most often, this is done with a sharp stick or pin. Reflexes will probably be tested using a reflex hammer as part of an assessment for nerve root damage. Although some of the nerve roots in the back don't result in lost reflexes when damaged, the classical finding of a "dropped" reflex in the ankle, in concert with other abnormalities, may indicate a specific nerve root arising from the back is damaged.

The practitioner may attempt to determine if there are signs of nerve root tension or compression by performing the straight-leg raise test. In this test, the patient is usually asked lie back on a table. This may be uncomfortable for you in the acute phases of back injury, so be sure to let your examiner know what movements or positions are especially painful. While you are lying on your back, the doctor or practitioner will ask you to relax while they gradually lift one leg, with the knee straight, bending at the hip. He or she should ask you to report if the movement becomes painful at any point but be sure to point out if much pain does occur and indicate where the pain is. Pain in the back of the leg can be just "tight hamstrings," but pain in the lower back that comes on suddenly as the leg is raised has classically been interpreted as supportive of nerve root injury. After the leg is raised to 90 degrees or to the point of maximum tolerable pain, the leg is gradually lowered and the test repeated on the opposite side. All the pieces of information from the examination should be interpreted together with the history you have provided during the visit and through other communications. As noted above, the most common presentation of nerve root injury is pain and weakness together but variations do occur and the exam is a way of sorting out the contributions of various back problems.

One twist in all of this is that nerve root injury often occurs as a result of damage to a disc, whether herniation, protrusion, or bulging tear. The damaged disc may itself be painful and will produce a pain that is more central in the back and may be acutely worse with the movements required to get into position for the straight leg raise test and other parts of the exam. This active overlay of disc pain on top of nerve root pain may be difficult for some less "pain expert" clinicians to sort out. Don't give up hope if your doctor doesn't immediately understand everything that's going on with your back. You may need to go to the next level and seek out more expert care, but make sure that if you have pain severe enough to stop you from going to work or school that you are actively looking for answers as to why it still hurts. The examination findings of nerve root injury can be subtle in some cases, especially if someone is confused about the overall picture of your pain.

The Explanation

The nerves that arise from the spinal cord stream downward as they spiral around to the front of the body from the back. When injured, the nerves send out pain signals that can be felt at some distance from where the injury actually is located in the back. The pain of an injured nerve can be deep and aching or electrical and shooting, or bizarrely painful and difficult to describe.

Radiating back pain is the classic description given to pain that is caused by a pinched nerve in the back. Typically, this is caused by a herniated disc, although other problems can produce these same symptoms. A herniated disc is the usual cause when symptoms come on suddenly and after a particular event: bending to lift, sneezing hard, jumping off from a height. A pain is called *radiating* when there is a component of the pain in one location and another, seemingly related pain nearby. In the case of the lower back pain due to a herniated disc and nerve compression, there may be one pain in the back and another component that extends down into the leg on that side. The first thing that leaps to the mind of most doctors when they hear about radiating back pain is the possibility of a nerve root compression due to a herniated disc. Although there are other causes of radiating back pain, such as compression of the sciatic nerve in the buttock, the classic association is with a pinched nerve due to a slipped disc.

Questions Your Doctor Will Ask

Does the pain in your leg extend below the knee? Pain below the knee is more often associated with the most common forms of nerve root compression. Pain that does not extend below the knee may mean there is a pinched nerve higher in the back, or that another problem is causing your pain.

(continued)

In most situations, back pain caused by a compressed nerve root in the back is very severe. Often described as eight on a scale of 10 or greater, the pain can take on one of several guises. The pain can begin with some subtleness, worsening progressively over a few days, or with a popping sensation while lifting and evolve fairly rapidly to an incapacitating severity. It can be fairly mild for a period and then suddenly worsen. The one thing these pains have in common is an element of pain in the back and an element of pain running down into the leg.

The precise location of radiating back pain in the leg will vary depending on which nerve root is endangered. There are several nerve roots arising from the lower part of the spine and each one of these nerves, when compressed, will produce a particular pattern of pain and limitations in function. The most common root to be damaged is the L5 root, the 5th lumbar root. This nerve comes out from the lower back, descends into the leg by passing deep through the buttock, and spirals around the back of the thigh to supply sensation to the top of the foot. If the nerve root is seriously compressed and functionally disabled by the pressure on it in the back, specific muscles will be weak—in this case, the muscles

Radiating pain ▶

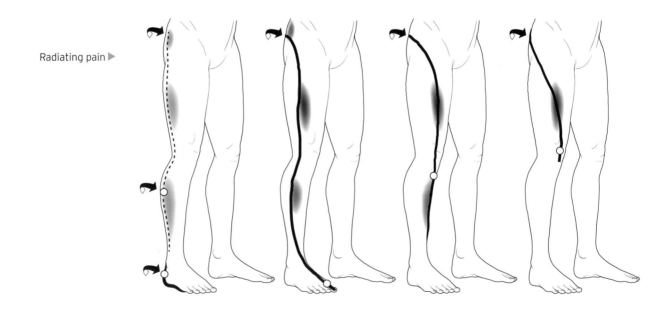

that control the lifting of the foot and the ability to turn the foot from side to side. Sometimes people with nerve damage at the L5 level will have difficulty with frequent tripping because this nerve controls the muscles that lift the front of the foot as we walk. Frequent toe catching can also result from damage to the L4 nerve root or to problems in other parts of the nervous system. When the S1 nerve root is damaged, people may have difficulty walking on toes. This may not be as noticeable but may lead to some fatigue with walking or some difficulties at reaching high objects where stretching up is required. Compression of the L3 nerve root can be more subtle to detect, as the pain may or may not extend below the knee and the weakness may be in the thigh muscles. Since L3 nerve root compression is less common, some physicians may not be as familiar with this pattern.

In some cases, when the pain is very severe or persistent, the person can actually perceive the pain as occurring partially in the opposite leg as well. This probably has to do with how the body handles profound pain signals with the overflow from one side spilling onto to the opposite side. Recent research indicates that the phenomenon of opposite side pain (contralateral pain) may be due to the activation of the glial cells that are present in the spinal cord. Normally, these glial cells provide much needed nutrient support to the nerve cells, but in certain situations, like profound pain, the glial cells can become abnormally activated, and this activation has been associated with pain spreading to the opposite limb. There are no medical treatment strategies currently targeting the glial cell activation process; however, it has been hypothesized that early, aggressive pain treatment may help prevent the changes leading to chronic pain states.

(Questions Your Doctor Will Ask continued)

Do you have a detectable area of numbness? You can test this using gentle pressure with a toothpick. Not everyone with nerve root compression will have an area of appreciable numbness. When numbness is present, you should alert your doctor to this so that he or she can investigate the pattern and see if this fits together with nerve root compression syndrome.

Do you have weakness in one or more specific leg muscles? People with nerve compression syndrome (radiculopathy) may have difficulty with one or more of the following:
• rising from a squat
• walking up on tip-toe
• walking on the heels

If you check these areas and notice that something doesn't seem right, be sure to notify your healthcare provider when you are seen. If you decide to try these maneuvers at home, make sure to have someone with you to provide support should you have any unsteadiness or difficulty.

CHAPTER RESOURCES

1. Freynhagen, R., R. Rolke, R. Baron, T.R. Tölle, A.K. Rutjes, S. Schu, and R.D. Treede. 2008. Pseudoradicular and radicular low-back pain—a disease continuum rather than different entities? Answers from quantitative sensory testing. *Pain* 135 (1-2): 65-74.

2. Bolton, J.E. and M.N. Christensen. 1994. Back pain distribution patterns: Relationship to subjective measures of pain severity and disability. *J Manipulative Physiol Ther* 17 (4): 211-8.

3. Gregory, D.S., et al. 2008. Acute lumbar disk pain: navigating evaluation and treatment choices. *American Family Physician* 78 (7): 835-42.

4. Selby, Anna. *Banish Back Pain the Pilates Way*. London: Thorsons, 2003.

5. McKenzie, Robin and Craig Kuby. *7 Steps To A Pain-Free Life: How To Rapidly Relieve Back and Neck Pain*. New York: Plume, 2001.

6. Cox, James. *Low Back Pain: Mechanism, Diagnosis and Treatment*. Baltimore: Lippincott Williams & Wilkins, 1999.

7. Hochschuler, Stephen and Bob Reznik. *Treat Your Back Without Surgery: The Best Non-Surgical Alternatives for Eliminating Back and Neck Pain*. Alameda, CA: Hunter House Inc., 2002.

8. McKenzie, Robin. *Treat Your Own Back*. Minneapolis, MN: Orthopedic Physical Therapy Products, 2006.

9. Brownstein, Art. *Healing Back Pain Naturally*. New York: Simon & Schuster, 2001.

10. Filler, Aaron. *Do You Really Need Back Surgery?* New York: Oxford University Press, 2004.

11. Larson, Sanford and Dennis Maiman. *Surgery of the Lumbar Spine*. New York: Thieme, 1999.

12. Lurie, J.D., S.C. Faucett, B. Hanscom, T.D. Tosteson, P.A. Ball, W.A. Abdu, J.W. Frymoyer, and J.N. Weinstein. 2008. Lumbar discectomy outcomes vary by herniation level in the Spine Patient Outcomes Research Trial. *J Bone Joint Surg Am*. 90 (9): 1811-9.

13. Dollinger, V., A.A. Obwegeser, M. Gabl, P. Lackner, M. Koller, and K. Galiano. 2008. Sporting activity following discectomy for lumbar disc herniation. *Orthopedics* 31 (8): 756.

14. Teli, M., A. Lovi, M. Brayda-Bruno, A. Zagra, A. Corriero, F. Giudici, and L. Minoia. 2010. Higher risk of dural tears and recurrent herniation with lumbar micro-endoscopic discectomy. *Eur Spine J* [Epub].

What is the difference between a disc bulge, a disc protrusion, and a herniated disc?

A disc bulge is a bulging out of a disc in such a way that there is no fundamental compromise of the ordinary relationship between the disc core (nucleus pulposus) and the tough exterior of the disc (annulus fibrosis). Disc bulges are incredibly common. There is no evidence to suggest that a disc bulge is necessarily painful, and a disc bulge alone, in the absence of other spine problems, should not result in a compressed nerve.

A disc protrusion is a focal pouching out of the nerve. In many instances, a disc protrusion is felt to represent a type of disc herniation in which the core of the disc has breached the tough outer ring, but has not extended through the ligament (posterior longitudinal ligament) that lies between the disc and the spinal canal. In some instances, a disc protrusion is a radiologist's term that is used when a disc bulge assumes a particular geometry such that the disc pouches out very sharply from the regular contours of the disc.

A disc herniation is an abnormal state in which the inner contents of the disc (nucleus pulposus) have pushed through the tough exterior of the disc. Whether the disc contents have pushed up to the posterior longitudinal ligament, pushed through the ligament, or burst through the ligament and separated from the disc proper determines whether the herniation will be described as a contained herniation, a disc extrusion, or a sequestered disc herniation, respectively. It is important to distinguish between the different forms of herniation as the treatments and likelihood of success will vary according to the diagnosis.

My doctor says I have a disc fragment. What is that?

Occasionally, the force of an injury that leads a disc to herniate is so great that a piece of the disc literally breaks off as the disc contents burst through the tough outer covering of the disc. This is referred to as a *disc fragment* or a *sequestered disc*. To visualize the difference, first imagine squeezing some toothpaste from a tube with your hands as you normally would. The ribbon of toothpaste usually stays attached to the tube until you stop squeezing and move your toothbrush away. Now imagine you took that same uncapped tube of toothpaste, placed it on the floor, and stomped hard with your foot. The toothpaste would fly out of the tube and a piece of the toothpaste would separate from the tube and the rest of the toothpaste. This is like a disc fragment; when it is separated from the rest of the disc, it can move around within the spinal canal, potentially lodging up against a nerve root and causing severe pain.

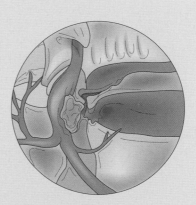

▲ Disc fragment or sequestered disc pushing on the nerve root.

CHAPTER 3

Torn and Painful Discs

Physical therapy, patience, and multiple medications are often necessary.

the **DIAGNOSIS**

> **Do you have pain located primarily in the mid-line (center) of the back?**

> **Does your pain seem to worsen with almost any activity?**

Pain that is most strongly felt in the center of the back (at the mid-line) and gets worse with sitting, standing, rising up, bending forward, or coughing and sneezing is usually due to disc injury. You may have a torn disc, especially if your pain started fairly suddenly after an accident, lifting something too heavy, or some other identifiable mishap.

Sometimes, disc pain relates to an accumulated injury and may be associated with damage to the top or bottom of the disc. In both of these situations, the pain can be mild-to-moderate when a person is resting the back, as when he or she lies still with the legs supported or with the body curled up in fetal position. This pain can suddenly get worse with standing or sitting, as pressure on the disc rises rapidly in these positions. If this sounds like your situation, you may have discogenic pain. Read on!

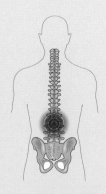

the PRESCRIPTION

Back pain due to a damaged disc presents special challenges and requires knowl-edgeable medical assessment and care. Because the disc is not a bony structure, it cannot be seen on X-ray, and for this reason, an MRI of the back will be needed as a first diagnostic test when disc problems are suspected. Disc pain can be expect-ed to have a much longer recovery course than pain due to simple muscle strain. Disc pain may respond to an intensive course of physical therapy and can even benefit from pain medicine injections.

If you have a torn disc (sometimes referred to as an annular disc tear):
- Your doctor should recommend physical therapy, especially if there is sub-stantial pain with movement.
    - Physical therapy can take a lot of effort. Especially after the first phases where the focus of therapy may be getting you more comfortable and reducing associated muscle spasm, you'll be expected to do specific exercises every day.
    - Sometimes physical therapy seems to make the pain a bit worse; this is part of the strengthening processes. Severe pain should be discussed with your doctor and therapist, but a certain amount of recuperation pain is to be expected.
- Your doctor should prescribe or recommend some medicine to control the pain.
    - Make sure that you understand the instructions for taking the medicine. When pain is limiting your ability to work, make sure you ask about taking the medicine "around the clock" or on a "time-contingent" basis rather than "as needed."
    - Be aware of potential side effects (bothersome symptoms that arise in people taking the medicine) as well as the potential for adverse events. Adverse events are more problematic than side effects; they will vary depending on the pain medicine used, and can include a risk of gastro-intestinal bleeding, severe constipation, or other problems.

- Your doctor may refer you to a pain medicine specialist, especially if there is a severe degree of pain that is not responding fully to medications that you take by mouth.
    - For an isolated disc tear with severe pain, injections can help.
        - Injection of medicine into the disc area is associated with improved pain control in the first weeks after injection.
        - Long-term effects are minimal; if you'd rather not have an injection, don't worry that your prospects for recovery are necessarily dimmer.
    - When a disc tear is part of a more complex back problem, injections can help define the components that are causing pain.

If you have a disrupted disc (sometimes referred to as *end-plate damage*):
- Your doctor may recommend physical therapy.
- Your doctor should prescribe or recommend some medicine to control the pain.
- Your doctor may recommend that you see an interventional pain medicine specialist because injections can sometimes help.
- In severe cases, your doctor may recommend a surgical evaluation.

The Good News

People with torn discs typically recover fully.

The process of recovery can leave you with a stronger, healthier back.

▶ A disc with a major tear. Note the torn edges of the disc and the disc core material pushing through.

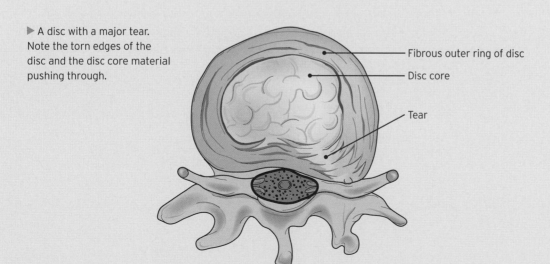

Fibrous outer ring of disc

Disc core

Tear

When to See a Physiatrist

Some doctors don't recognize disc tears as a potential source of strong pain, and they may dismiss the report of these findings in the MRI report. If your back hurts a lot and your doctor says there's nothing wrong, make sure you have copies of all your back images and the reports of those, then find a provider who is very knowledgeable about back problems. Often times, physical medicine and rehabilitation specialists known as *physiatrists* are especially attuned to problems relating to injury and repair of the spine.

WHAT IF YOUR DOCTOR DIAGNOSES A BULGING DISC?

In this case, physical therapy and exercise are usually best. Bulging discs have been reported to be very common in the normal, "pain-free" population. Nonetheless, people vary greatly in the degree of pain they may experience for a particular problem. If your doctor reports that a bulging disc is the only thing wrong with your back and you still cannot function properly due to back pain, you may want to look elsewhere for answers and support.

As long as you don't have any of the red flags (see Chapter 1) of back pain, it's usually okay to pursue a course of back strengthening and stretching. Physical therapy isn't likely to produce lasting damage and can result in a stronger back that puts less pressure on an irritated disc. You may want to read through the second half of this book where lifestyle choices for a better back are covered in detail.

WHAT IF YOUR DOCTOR FINDS THAT YOU HAVE DISC DEGENERATION?

As the back ages, the discs gradually become less spongy and resilient. This is not necessarily associated with pain, and in fact may reduce the chances that a disc will be herniated when subjected to strong stresses. A severely degenerated disc can be associated with pain, whether due to chronic inflammation (arthritis), a loss of the disc height leading to nerve root compression, or chronic activation of pain fibers in the area. There are some cases where a degenerated disc is severe enough to warrant surgical intervention. Degeneration of the spine is covered in more detail in Chapter 11.

In rare cases, central back pain may be due to a mass (tumor), an infection (abcess), or a spinal malformation. These causes of central back pain are readily assessed through MRI and the other diagnostic tests that are widely used. The treatment for these conditions is individualized.

▶ Cutaway view of the spine showing the location of the vertebral endplate relative to the disc core and the outer ring of the disc.

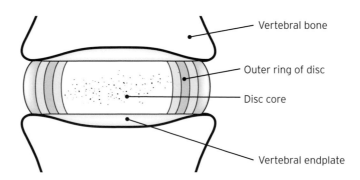

Vertebral bone

Outer ring of disc

Disc core

Vertebral endplate

The Treatment

When your doctor recommends physical therapy, realize that this is a wonderful part of modern medicine. Most physical therapists are drawn to this work through an intense desire to promote human health and fitness. Several different kinds of treatment are included in the realm of physical therapy that will be useful for the treatment of vertebral disc problems: thermal therapies, manual therapies, electrical stimulation therapies, traction/inversion therapies, and conditioning and strengthening.

THERMAL THERAPIES ARE HOT AND COLD

Although we traditionally think of using ice during the first forty-eight hours after an injury, ice continues to be a useful part of pain control and improves outcomes with physical therapy. Because your physical therapy program will progress to exercises that will push your muscles to new levels of strength and performance, ice may be used at the end of sessions. Icing then will help reduce the pain of muscle strain and stress on the disc as you are working on the strengthening and conditioning parts of the physical therapy program. If your physical therapist is not offering ice at the end of each session and you think it would be helpful, go ahead and ask. The best physical therapists are open to suggestions and will check with your doctor about this if necessary.

MANUAL THERAPIES REDUCE PRESSURE ON THE DISC

One way that manual therapy can help is by addressing the position and alignment of the vertebrae. Although not all physical therapists are skilled in this area, some have the capacity to make gentle adjustments to the spine and improve the alignment of the vertebral column. This can really relieve the pressure on a disc as the bones are coaxed back into their proper relative positions. Another way that manual therapy can help is by addressing the profound muscle spasms that frequently accompany disc damage.

ELECTRICAL STIMULATION THERAPY IS WIDELY ACCEPTED

In this technique, small, rapid electrical impulses are transmitted to the body through "sticky-pad" electrodes. These electrical impulses can cause the muscle to relax, which may loosen some of the pressure on the disc that nearby muscles in spasm can produce. Because the injured disc signals pain to the spinal cord, and this can result in a reflex signal to neighboring muscles to contract, muscle spasm is a frequent accompaniment to disc-related pain.

TRACTION AND INVERSION THERAPIES ARE HELPFUL

With traction, the disc will bulge less, and the resting pressure on the disc will be lowered, potentially relieving pain. Traction can range from milder forms that involve putting the legs up on a triangular bolster to more aggressive forms, which require the use of weights and even belts. Inversion therapy can be very effective in reducing painful pressures on injured discs. There are different approaches to using inversion in a physical therapy regimen. (See Chapter 20.)

STRENGTHENING AND CONDITIONING ARE MAINSTAYS

There are many great exercises to help strengthen the back muscles. Your physical therapist can guide you through a sequence that is most appropriate to your back and pain level. A good place to start after a disc injury is by doing the pelvic tilt exercise. In this exercise, you strengthen the anterior abdominal muscles that are so critical to supporting the spine. You begin by lying on the back with the hips flexed and the knees bent. Gently at first, but gradually more strongly, tighten the abdominal muscles as you roll the front of the pelvis toward the chest. If you are having strong back pain, this movement may need to be very gentle at first; an almost subtle change in position may be all that is possible without increasing the pain. Hold this pelvic tilt for three seconds and then relax. Repeat this five times on the first day, but increase the length of hold and the number of repetitions each day.

ADVANTAGES AND DISADVANTAGES TO PHYSICAL THERAPY

Keep in mind that physical therapy is very effective for many types of back trouble, especially problems relating to discs. One great advantage of physical therapy is that it can turn the focus of your attention away from what is wrong and gradually improve your ability to do the things you enjoy. By reducing the need for medication over the long-term, physical therapy can help you avoid the awful side effects of most pain medications: mental cloudiness, memory loss, sleepiness, constipation, and sexual dysfunction. In fact, increased physical activity can help improve mood, memory, and sleep!

On the down side, physical therapy does frequently result in a temporary increase in pain or discomfort. If you're having a lot of pain after PT, make sure to let your therapist know. It's normal to feel like you've worked hard in physical therapy, and sometimes it's okay to feel a bit more pain in the first day or two after a physical therapy session. If your back pain is bad enough to interfere with activities at work or home, you should seek some physical therapy and expect to work hard on your way to getting great results.

Pain Medication Injections

If you are referred to an interventional pain specialist right away, chances are that your doctor thinks an injection of pain medication may be helpful to getting you back on track. The injection of pain medication into the area of an injured disc is a well-established pain medicine technique that can be very helpful for the immediate relief of pain.

The limitations of this approach are that in many cases, the injection will not result in lasting improvements, and clinical trials have suggested that the effects on long-term function cannot be proven. Moreover, these pain injections cannot be repeated over and over. This is because, in addition to local anesthetic—which provides immediate pain relief but wears off over the course of a day or two— most pain injections also include a long or intermediate-acting steroid. The steroid is helpful in terms of providing pain relief over the days to weeks that follow the injection. The problem is that steroids, when given repeatedly, have been associated with problems like abscess formation, diabetes, osteoporosis, and worse. For these reasons, a pain injection for disc injury is best used as a bridging strategy to get a person over a rough patch, pain-wise. It is not a long-term solution. Nonetheless, if the pain is unbearable and is interfering with your ability to function, getting some immediate pain relief is valuable as a goal.

NERVE-DESTROYING CHEMICALS WORK TEMPORARILY

The injection of nerve-destroying chemicals into an area is intended to disrupt the pain-sensing fibers and block pain signals arising from an injured or irritated area in the back. The problem with this approach is that nerves will almost always grow back and sometimes more painfully so than before. The long-term outcomes of patients receiving injections of nerve-destroying chemicals for pain have indicated that pain problems may be better temporarily, but often return worse than ever over the ensuing few months.

What's New: The European Gastro-Protective View

The primary limitation of using NSAIDs is the occurrence of serious problems in the digestive tract, including bleeding from the stomach and intestines. The number of people who experience life-threatening bleeding with the use of NSAIDs is believed to be much higher in the U.S. than in Europe. The reason for this is thought to be the widespread use of "gastro-protective" medications in combination with NSAIDs in Europe. Because the phenomenon of bleeding from the stomach is so common with NSAIDs, some doctors have adopted the strategy of always prescribing a medicine to protect the stomach whenever NSAIDs are prescribed.

Your doctor may recommend that you take ibuprofen with meals. In Europe, they go one step further and instruct patients to take an acid-reducing medication at the time of using NSAIDs. Examples of these medications might include ranitidine (Zantac), cimetidine (Tagamet), or Omeprazole (Prilosec). Some of these medicines are now available over the counter, meaning they can be obtained without a prescription.

(continued)

SPINAL CORD STIMULATION MASKS PAIN WITH A BUZZ

If your disc-related pain problem is very chronic and painful, your doctor may speak with you about a spinal cord stimulator trial. The spinal cord stimulator is a high-tech approach to a persistent pain problem. It requires the placement of a precision-engineered electrical contact strip on the posterior surface of the spine. To be effective, the stimulator strip must be positioned over the spinal cord in just the right place to block the pain signal from reaching the brain. For this reason, spinal cord stimulators are first "trialed" before permanently placed.

While the spinal cord stimulator can be very effective in reducing the sensation of pain, it does nothing to correct the underlying problem with the back. When the stimulator is correctly positioned and turn on, most people will feel a buzzing or tingling sensation in place of their usual pain. Although the buzzing can feel rather distracting at first, it is much preferable to the sensation of strong pain.

The strip electrode is connected via wires tunneled under the skin to a control unit that is often located just under the skin in the lower abdomen. The control unit contains batteries and a programmable control element. Working with a trained specialist, a person who has a spinal cord stimulator can progressively change the settings to fine-tune the area of coverage (the part of the body that perceives the buzzing) as well as changing the stimulus program by increasing or decreasing the intensity and pattern of electrical signals to the stimulator's contact strip. Although many patients report dramatic pain relief with the spinal cord stimulator, it is often the case that some pain medication will still be required for optimal pain control. The advantage is that pain control is often better overall after the stimulator and even if medications continue, doses are often lower, leading to fewer side effects.

Taking Medications by Mouth

Disc-related pain can be very strong in the first several weeks after an injury. What distinguishes disc-related pain from an ordinary muscle strain is the much, much longer time that is required for most people to recover from a disc injury. Muscle strain typically lasts a few days; disc pain can last three to four months in the more severe cases. In addition, the pain due to a disc injury typically relates to the degree of inflammation that occurs after a disc injury. Although some inflammation is needed for healing, the usual experience is that controlling inflammation will speed recovery and decrease pain. For this reason, it is usually necessary to take medications that control both inflammation and pain after disc injury; more than one medication may be needed.

NSAIDS BLOCK PAIN SIGNALS

One mainstay of treatment for disc-related back pain is the non-steroidal anti-inflammatory drug, or NSAID. NSAIDs are valuable medications because they both block pain signaling and can reduce the body's inflammatory responses to the injury. A broad class of drugs, NSAIDs have been widely used by millions and millions of people.[1] Although there are rare cases of allergy and drug reactions, for most people these medicines are extremely effective at reducing pain, and when used properly, are quite safe. The best known NSAID is ibuprofen, sold as Advil and Motrin.

Ibuprofen is a very effective pain-reducing medication. Available at your pharmacy, ibuprofen comes in 200 mg tablets. The recommended dosage for an adult is usually two tablets. There are important guidelines for using this medication of the bottle, so please read the fine print. At the 400 mg dose, the medication is expected to relieve pain for four to six hours. This can mean that you'd get partway through a night's sleep and wake up in pain. Another factor is the weight or size of the person taking the medicine. A person weighing 110 lbs will get more benefit from this dosage than a 240-lb person. You should discuss with your healthcare provider whether ibuprofen is the best medicine for you. In some cases, physicians will prescribe a stronger dose of ibuprofen, but remember, the more medication, the more side effects. The higher doses, while potentially more effective, will increase the risk for gastrointestinal bleeding. You should not fill a prescription for high-strength ibuprofen without understanding your gastro-protective strategy.

Another NSAID gaining popularity is naproxen, which is sold under several names including Naprosyn and Aleve. Your doctor can prescribe this medication, but it is now available over the counter as well. This medicine is used at doses that begin around 200 mg. For many people, this medication is very effective against pain, and it has the advantage that pain relief may last longer, perhaps six to eight hours. You doctor can prescribe longer-lasting NSAIDs or medications that have a different side-effect profile. In some cases, a physician will choose to prescribe opioids for back pain.

You will need to communicate clearly and calmly with your healthcare provider about your pain. If you feel like you're being ignored, patronized, or belittled, try to find another provider who will listen to your report of pain. If you really do have a disc injury, the recovery course can stretch out over several weeks and sometimes a few months. You don't want to be in more than mild pain for that long a period. Sometimes making a pain calendar or a daily log of your pain in-

(Whats New? continued)

Although it's sometimes uncomfortable to think about taking two medicines when only one is *really needed*, evidence indicates that Europeans are very successful in preventing the bleeding complications of NSAIDs, whereas estimates are that 30,000 Americans each year require medical attention for gastrointestinal bleeding due to NSAIDs! Make sure you discuss both NSAIDs and anti-ulcer (gastro-protective) medications with your doctor.

Warning! For Those at Risk for Heart and Kidney Disease

NSAIDs are associated with a small increase in the risk of heart attack and acute kidney failure.[2,3] Both of these effects are very, very small at ordinary doses of these medicines, but if you are at risk for heart disease or have a family history of kidney disease, you should discuss these concerns with your doctor so that an informed decision can be made. You may want to learn more by visiting the American Heart Association's website for patients: www.hearthub.org. If you have high blood pressure, a risk factor for both heart disease and kidney disease, you should discuss NSAIDs with your doctor before starting a course of therapy with these medicines.

tensity, recorded on a zero-to-ten scale, can be a helpful communication tool and may illustrate what you're going through to someone who would otherwise have difficulty understanding how serious the problem really is.

MULTIPLE MEDICATIONS MAY BE NECESSARY

The pain of a disc injury may be due to multiple mechanisms: one relating to the actual pain-sensing of the injury, one related to the inflammation that results as your body tries to repair the disc, and one related to the response of the nearby nerves to the release of nerve-irritating substances which may have been release from the disc at the time of injury. For this reason, it is very important to recognize that more than one medication may be needed to control the pain. People with disc injuries may require one medicine to help reduce the inflammation-related component of pain (an NSAID, for example), one medicine to help control the pain (sometimes an NSAID, sometimes another medication), and one medicine to reduce the neuropathic pain, if any is present (a medication such as gabapentin, for example). Although it's always better to keep to one medicine for a problem if one is enough, there are usually multiple aspects contributing to pain after disc injury, and multiple medicines may be appropriate. Make sure to discuss this with your doctor or other healthcare provider.

Testing For Disc Injury

Some doctors may resist ordering an MRI, as they have been taught that all back pain not associated with demonstrable nerve root damage is best treated by ordering the least number of tests and by dispensing more pain killers. The problem with this approach is that it does not recognize the very special needs of patients with disc problems.

MRI PLAYS AN IMPORTANT ROLE IN DIAGNOSIS

Magnetic Resonance Images have been very helpful in clarifying the nature of disc injury. In fact, MRI is essential for defining disc injury as a cause of back pain. One well-researched study concluded that it was impossible to make the diagnosis of disc injury on clinical exam alone and that MRI was required.[4]

The value of Magnetic Resonance Imaging (MRI) in guiding the treatment of people with low back pain has been dramatically downplayed in the medical literature. Disc pain is terribly intense for many, if not most, people. It takes an exceptionally long time to recover from new disc pain, and MRI is quite good at detecting new disc damage. In fact, a 1992 study showed that MRI very selectively identified people with disc damage (few false-positive results) and was very powerful in terms of predicting severe disc damage. The real limitation may be that many doctors are not properly educated about recognizing disc-related back problems—they may not have had more than one or two hours of education about spine problems in all four years of medical school!

If you have back pain, getting an MRI can be the difference between night and day. By identifying a significant disc problem, you can anticipate a much longer recovery course that will require more intensive efforts at pain control and more physical therapy. If you don't have an MRI and you actually do have an injured disc, you will most likely have substantial pain that takes a long time to improve; however, you won't have a lot of physical evidence to prove that you have a real problem. You may experience pressure from your employer, your health insurer, and others to get back to work. Because disc injuries can take weeks and sometimes months to heal, you will be faced with a very difficult situation trying to defend your pain as real and possibly being pressured to make choices that will interfere with speedy and full recovery. If your doctor fails to recognize the true nature of the problem, you may end up with a denied claim for short-term disability coverage, or worse yet, out of a job.[5]

PROVACATIVE DISCOGRAPHY IS A MORE INVASIVE TEST FOR PAIN

Provacative discography is a test wherein a small catheter-needle is placed into the core of the disc using fluoroscopic (multi-directional, low-intensity X-ray) guidance. Once positioning of the catheter-needle in the disc core is confirmed with dye, tracer is injected into the disc under pressure. The pressure is quite intense and is intended to stress the disc, partially simulating the pressures of bending and lifting. If this pressurization of the disc causes pain that is like the pain the patient normally feels, it will be labeled "concordant pain." For the test to be truly diagnostic, however, the doctor performing the test must also place the catheter-needle into at least one other disc in the back and pressurize that disc. If that disc is normal, it should not reproduce the pain that is usually felt.

What We Don't Know: Recovery Times After Disc Injury

There is no definitive study describing the time course of recovery after a disc tear or a diagnosis of internal disc disruption. As with any study, there are limits, but better information about what to expect in the recovery course from disc injury would be most welcome. Stay tuned!

Tracer is used in these injections because it allows the doctor to also make an assessment of the physical integrity of the disc. If dye stays contained within the core of the disc, then the disc structure is normal. If dye begins to leak out and demonstrates cracks, tears, or ruptures of the disc structures, this is supportive of internal disc disruption as a diagnosis. Part of this study is expected to somewhat painful, but it should occur in a controlled setting and any severe pain should be reported to the staff immediately. For the test to be most helpful, those present should not tell the patient which disc is being tested prior to putting pressure into the system, as this could influence the outcome of the test.[6]

The Explanation

Central back pain that worsens with standing or pressure on the back is the classic description given to pain caused by an injured vertebral disc. Most often, central back pain is a challenge because the limitations on how much a person can move without provoking pain can be very constraining. For most people, it's impossible to work a normal schedule if every time you sit or stand for more than five minutes, your back begins to scream out in pain.

ANATOMY OF A DISC

The vertebral disc is a sometimes tough, sometimes resilient structure in the back that is central to making the spine both flexible and strong. However, the disc is subjected to many pressures and strains, especially when heavy objects are lifted or when accidental injury occurs. A disc that is injured or damaged by tearing at the edge can push into the adjacent vertebral bone, causing damage there. Although the center of the disc does not contain pain fibers, the edges are richly innervated and pain fibers can proliferate after injury, making the chronically stressed disc more susceptible. The damaged disc can become extremely painful, but taking the right steps can improve your chances of making peace with it.

THE RESILIENT DISC CORE

The central core of the disc, or nucleus pulposus, is designed for durable resilience. It is made up of a spongy, gelatin-like substance. Although the gel-like center of the disc functions very well early in life, over time the disc core desiccates or dries out. This desiccation process is considered normal. On MRI scans, it is possible for the radiologist to observe this drying out of the disc. Desiccated discs are thought to be more resistant to herniation but presumably the other forms of disc damage such as tears, dislocations, and internal disc disruption are even more likely. Disc desiccation is thought to be an irreversible process, and the center of the disc does not regenerate as far as we know. The core of the disc does not contain any blood vessels and does not have any nerves: it is understood that the gel-like filling of the disc is a hostile environment for living structures such as nerves and blood vessels.

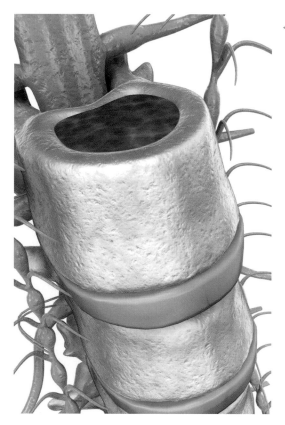

◀ Cut-away view of the spine showing a vertebral endplate

THE DISC'S OUTER RING

The outer part of the disc is a tough fibrous ring called the *annulus fibrosus*. Composed of many layers of strong collagen, the annulus complex serves to flexibly connect adjacent vertebral bones and contain the disc core material (nucleus pulposus).[7] Unlike the disc core, the annulus contains blood vessels and nerves, usually just in the outermost portion. The blood vessels and nerves are important for delivering nutrients to the annulus, allowing for sensations to be perceived from the area, and providing the capacity for repair. Evidence suggests that when discs are chronically damaged, the nerves in the outermost portion will sprout inward, growing toward the center of the disc. Unfortunately, nerves that sprout are predominantly of the pain-sensing variety. This in-growth of pain-sensing fibers after excessive chronic back strain may explain why some people have discs that are especially painful following injury while others seem to bounce back quickly after the same experience.[8] It may also be that over time, if the back has a chance to recuperate properly, the pain-sensing nerve fibers may die back to their original locations and the back may once again become more robust against various insults such as riding horses, riding in the back of a school bus, or bouncing along the back of a pick-up truck.

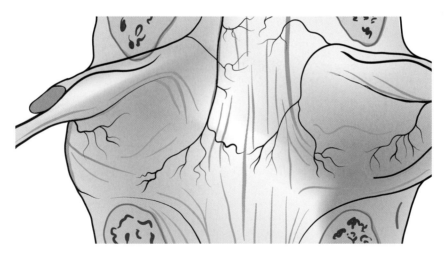

▲ Nerves reaching into the disc

The outer part of the disc, unlike the core, has a capacity for repair after injury, although this capacity is quite limited and oftentimes seems to advance very slowly.[9] The capacity of the disc's outer ring to repair is, in practical terms, restricted to injuries that involve annular tears. (More serious injuries, like those resulting in disc herniations, may require surgical intervention.) An annular tear is a rip in the fibrous-ring that surrounds the disc core. Often, the tear in the annulus is limited to the outer portion, as if the outermost fibers had ripped or torn from the stress placed on the spine at the time of injury. Under some circumstances, multiple tears are located in one or more discs. Sometimes, the disc's ring can tear in such a way that the innermost fibers of the ring separate from the outermost fibers. The repair process in the disc takes weeks to months to complete; during that time, the back will not be as strong as it is ordinarily, and the person with the disc injury may experience high levels of pain and may even experience pain that extends down into the leg.[10]

THE DISC-ENDPLATE

The disc-endplate is the place where the top or bottom of the disc connects to the vertebral bone above or below the disc. In recent years, the vertebral end-plate has come to be recognized as an important location of disc disruption and potential cause of pain.[11] The disc-endplate can essentially shatter (like a window in a blast zone) when a disc is suddenly pressurized. The endplate is a structure with both blood vessels and nerves, and so the response to injury includes swelling, pain, placement of repair tissue, and ultimately re-establishment of a durable solid structure.[12] Damage to endplates is readily visible on MRI and these damage-related alternations have been called *modic changes*. Studies of people with back pain and those without pain have shown that disc bulges are not likely to be a cause of pain for many people.[13] End-plate changes, however, are associated with pain for many people and like disc tears may take a long period to repair.

CHAPTER RESOURCES

1. World Health Organization (WHO). "WHO Model List of Essential Medicines," http://whqlibdoc.who.int/hq/2005/a87017_eng.pdf. March 2005.

2. Lafrance, J.P. and D.R. Miller. 2009. Selective and non-selective non-steroidal anti-inflammatory drugs and the risk of acute kidney injury. *Pharmacoepidemiology and Drug Safety* 18:923-931.

3. Van Staa, T.P., S. Rietbrock, E. Setakis, and H.G. Leufkens. 2008. Does the varied use of NSAIDs explain the differences in the risk of myocardial infarction? *Journal of Internal Medicine* 264: 481-92.

4. Schwarzer, A.C., C.N. Aprill, R. Derby, J. Fortin, G. Kine, and N. Bogduk. 1995. The prevalence and clinical features of internal disc disruption in patients with chronic low back pain. *Spine (Phila Pa 1976)* 20 (17): 1878-83.

5. Aprill, C. and N. Bogduk. 1992. High-intensity zone: A diagnostic sign of painful lumbar disc on magnetic resonance imaging. *Br J Radiol* 65 (773): 361-9.

6. Schwarzer, A.C., C.N. Aprill, R. Derby, J. Fortin, G. Kine, and N. Bogduk. 1995. The prevalence and clinical features of internal disc disruption in patients with chronic low back pain. *Spine (Phila Pa 1976)* 20 (17): 1878-83.

7. Gruber, H.E., J. Ingram, K. Leslie, and E.N. Hanley Jr. 2008. Gene expression of types I, II, and VI collagen, aggrecan, and chondroitin-6-sulfotransferase in the human annulus: In situ hybridization findings. *Spine J* 8 (5): 810-7.

8. Schellhas, K.P., S.R. Pollei, C.R. Gundry, and K.B. Heithoff. 1996. Lumbar disc high-intensity zone: Correlation of magnetic resonance imaging and discography. *Spine (Phila Pa 1976)* 21 (1): 79-86.

9. Yeung, A.T. and C.A. Yeung. 2006. In-vivo endoscopic visualization of patho-anatomy in painful degenerative conditions of the lumbar spine. *Surg Technol Int* 15: 243-56.

10. Peng, B., W. Wu, Z. Li, J. Guo, and X. Wang. 2007. Chemical radiculitis. *Pain* 127 (1-2): 11-6.

11. Jensen, T.S., J. Karppinen, J.S. Sorensen, J. Niinimäki, and C. Leboeuf-Yde. 2008. Vertebral endplate signal changes (Modic change): A systematic literature review of prevalence and association with non-specific low back pain. *Eur Spine J.* 17 (11): 1407-22.

12. Moore, R.J. 2006. The vertebral endplate: disc degeneration, disc regeneration. *European Spine Journal*. Vol. 15, Suppl. 3.

13. Rahmea, R. and R. Moussaa. 2008. The modic vertebral endplate and marrow changes: Pathologic significance and relation to low back pain and segmental instability of the lumbar spine. *American Journal of Neuroradiology* 29:838-842.

14. Schwarzer, A.C., C.N. Aprill, R. Derby, J. Fortin, G. Kine, and N. Bogduk. 1995. The prevalence and clinical features of internal disc disruption in patients with chronic low back pain. *Spine (Phila Pa 1976)* 20 (17): 1878-83.

What if my doctor doesn't want to take an MRI of my back?

In a landmark study of disc damage, researchers looked at the question of how to diagnose internal disc disruption. They found that this was a cause of 40 percent of low back pain in their study population. They further concluded that none of the clinical tests (tests your doctor could do in the exam room) could distinguish between people with this problem and those without it. If your back pain is severe enough to keep you from your work for more than a few days, you may need an MRI to solidify the diagnosis and effectively guide treatment.[14]

Is there anything else I can add to my daily routine to speed the healing of my injured disc?

There is some evidence to suggest that the dietary supplement glucosamine/chondroitin sulfate may be helpful for reducing inflammatory pain. This is discussed in more detail in Chapter 21. The exact mechanism by which glucosamine and chondroitin sulfate act to reduce inflammatory pain is not known and for some, the efficacy of these compounds is questionable. There is little evidence to support the ingestion of glucosamine/chondroitin sulfate in the absence of serious arthritis pain or inflammation, and routine usage is not something I recommend to patients. It is important to obtain all dietary supplements from a reputable manufacturer as the production of these is not as tightly regulated as the preparation of actual medications. Glucosamine/chondroitin sulfate tablets are fairly expensive and a course of therapy may cost more than twenty dollars.

CHAPTER 4

Sciatic and Other Nerve Compressions

Simple stretching exercises can resolve

mild cases and prevent relapses.

the DIAGNOSIS

> Do you have pain that starts in the buttock and runs down the back of the leg?

> Does your pain seem to get worse the longer you sit but ease off with standing and walking around?

Pain that runs down the back of the thigh and extends into the buttock and diffusely into the foot can be due to compression or irritation of the sciatic nerve. The sciatic nerve, the largest in the body, is prone to compression deep in the buttock; this pain is usually worse with prolonged sitting. There are actually several different syndromes of nerve compression that can occur in the back, buttock, or leg. Because sciatic nerve compression is most common, it is discussed first. Pudendal neuropathy, diabetic amyotrophy, post-herpetic neuralgia, and other causes of nerve pain are described later in this chapter. Each of these has symptoms particular to the nerve compressed, but the features of the pain may be similar. (Nerve root compression at the spinal level is described in Chapter 2.)

The diagnosis of sciatic nerve compression is made based on your medical history, findings in the physical exam, and possibly imaging or even electrical studies. Your doctor may perform some physical testing that is uncomfortable. If any of the tests provokes strong pain, make sure to speak up and let the doctor know what you're feeling. The doctor may bend your legs and apply pressure. In some cases, an examiner may press deeply into the buttock, trying to determine if there is appreciable muscle tightness or deep tenderness there. If the problem is very severe or lingers despite treatment, imaging or electrical testing becomes more likely.

Nerve compression pain is particularly distressing. It can be burning, deeply aching, or stabbing and producing electrical shocks. If you have pain that has electrical shocks from time to time, this is a strong indicator that nerve damage is part of the problem.

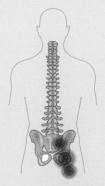

Sciatic Nerve Compression

Sciatic nerve compression is sometimes labeled *sciatica*, but that's not entirely correct. *Sciatica* is a term that originated in the fifteenth century and was used at that time to describe pain in the hip. It has been used for many years to describe pain that is primarily experienced down the back of the leg.[1] It is a broad umbrella term like the words *headache* or *depression*, which actually encompass many specific medical conditions.

The medical causes of sciatica as a syndrome of back, buttock, and leg pain include compression of the 4th or 5th lumbar nerve roots in the back, compression of other nerve roots, problems with the sacroiliac joint, and compression of the sciatic nerve as it courses from the spine into the leg. The most common location for the sciatic nerve to be compressed outside of the spinal cord is the place where it runs between two muscles deep in the buttock. Compression of the sciatic nerve in this location is frequently called *piriformis syndrome*.[2,3] It often occurs in the setting of trauma: car accidents, falls, and skiing accidents are examples. Although piriformis syndrome is rather common, it is often overlooked in medical school to the extent that the diagnosis is typically first suggested by the physical therapist rather than the doctor!

PINCHED NERVE

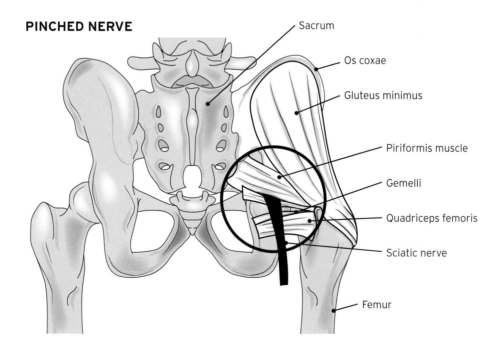

Sacrum

Os coxae

Gluteus minimus

Piriformis muscle

Gemelli

Quadriceps femoris

Sciatic nerve

Femur

the PRESCRIPTION

A first episode of sciatic nerve compression as a cause of back, buttock, and leg pain will require expert medical assessment and care. If you've had sciatic nerve compression before, be aware that it can flare up again, but you can sometimes treat a mild second episode with some simple stretching exercises.[4]

If you have sciatic nerve compression (sometimes called *piriformis syndrome*):
- Your doctor should recommend physical therapy, especially if pain is interfering with your activity level.
    - Physical therapy is exactly the right treatment for piriformis syndrome. The key to beating this problem is reducing associated muscle spasm. You'll be expected to do specific exercises every day.
    - Sometimes physical therapy may temporarily make the pain a bit worse. If you have more than a temporary increase in pain, let your doctor know.
- Your doctor may prescribe or recommend some medicine to control the pain, including over-the-counter pain relievers or, if nighttime pain is especially prominent, some prescription medications that are active against nerve pain.

If you have pudendal nerve compression (associated more with genital region pain):
- Your doctor may recommend physical therapy, especially if pain is interfering with your activity level.
    - Physical therapy for pudendal neuropathy is usually carried out by specially trained therapists. The delicate nature of the structures in the lower buttock and genital areas necessitates extra training and special techniques.
    - Sometimes injection or surgery is required. The pudendal nerve compression syndrome is not due to muscle spasm so much as to the development of fibrosis in the ligaments and other structures that the nerve passes by as it travels from the spine to the pelvis. These typically need to be released by a surgeon who has special experience with this problem.[5]

Warning! How to Prevent a Worsening of the Condition

Your physical therapist should make an assessment of your body mechanics and help you become aware of how to avoid worsening piriformis syndrome. The simple things include making sure that when you sit, your body is positioned symmetrically in front of your workstation. Make sure to get up and move around every 30 minutes or so if possible. Avoid carrying a heavy wallet in your back pocket. And learn how to strengthen and exercise the muscle that complements the function of piriformis. This will help to take some of the stress off of the piriformis muscle.

WHAT IF YOUR DOCTOR REFERS YOU TO A PAIN SPECIALIST OR WANTS TO DO AN INJECTION FOR PIRIFORMIS SYNDROME?

Piriformis syndrome is occasionally treated with injections to release the muscle. In most cases, however, the physical therapist's application of manual muscle-release treatments, electrical stimulation treatments, and stretching exercises will be sufficient. Be aware that anytime an injection is performed, there is a risk of not only infection, but longer-term damage and scarring to the muscle or nerve. This might convert a short-term problem into something more problematic.

WHAT IF YOUR DOCTOR RECOMMENDS SURGERY FOR SCIATIC NERVE COMPRESSION?

Surgery is only rarely considered for piriformis syndrome and is usually reserved for the most treatment-resistant forms of the condition. Surgery for piriformis syndrome can involve efforts to free up the nerve or to cut a fibrotic band that seems to be pressing on the nerve.

WHAT IF YOUR DOCTOR DIAGNOSES A THORACIC NERVE ROOT PROBLEM SUCH AS NERVE COMPRESSION, NERVE INJURY (NEUROPATHY), OR POST-HERPETIC NEURALGIA?

In this case, medication therapy is usually the first-line treatment. Depending on the specific problem, other treatments may be tried. If there is a nerve compression in the thoracic spine area, surgery or injection-type approaches are sometimes needed.

The Treatment

When your doctor recommends physical therapy, be confident that physical therapy is the best treatment available for piriformis syndrome.[6] Most physical therapists are very familiar with sciatic nerve compression and piriformis syndrome. Because piriformis syndrome is driven by muscle spasm in a particular muscle, the physical therapists are well equipped to treat this using multiple methods including thermal therapies, manual therapy, electrical stimulation, body awareness training, and stretching. Less commonly, injections of medications may offer temporary relief, and rarely surgery is needed for completely debilitating or structural problems.

PHYSICAL THERAPY RELAXES THE MUSCLE

The greatest aspect of physical therapy is the attitude that most physical therapists bring to their work: What you do makes a difference. Working with a qualified physical therapist will help you to remind yourself everyday that you can take steps to make this better and then follow through on those positive actions. The primary goal of physical therapy treatment is to relax the piriformis muscle so that the sciatic nerve can begin to function normally and stop signaling pain.

THERMAL THERAPIES PROVIDE IMMEDIATE RELIEF

Warm therapy can relax the muscles, while cold therapy blocks pain signals and reduces inflammation. Your therapist may use one or both of these approaches. She may also use ultrasound, which can create a gentle warming sensation deeper in the body. The warm packs that therapists use can only penetrate so far, and the piriformis muscle is actually pretty deep in the buttock, situated underneath the gluteus muscles. Ultrasound can be tuned to reach to varying depths in the body and may produce warming in structures that are too deep for access by warm compresses.

MANUAL THERAPY IS ESSENTIAL

Yes, it may be uncomfortable and feel a little awkward to have someone pressing their thumbs firmly into your buttock muscles, but this may be necessary. There is a wealth of clinical experience to support the use of trigger point massage for the relaxation of specific muscles.[7] A skilled manual therapist, whether doctor, nurse, physical therapist, or other person, can identify muscle spasm in the piriformis muscle and use their hands to relieve the spasm. Generally speaking, the location of the piriformis muscle prevents people from reaching this muscle manually, however.

Clair Davies has suggested a number of innovative ways that you can perform your own trigger-point therapy on hard-to-reach muscles.[8] Davies has had an interesting career path, as he started out as a piano tuner and only later in life became interested in healthcare. It seems that his experience tuning pianos has given him a special awareness of the dynamic tension that exists in the human body as muscles, nerves, and bones work together to create an integrated loco-motor system. His book on trigger points has become widely used and recommended because of the straightforward explanations involved and self-empowering approach that Davies encourages throughout. Because trigger points are hyper-responsive to direct stimulation and because they release inflammatory signals, it is important to combine trigger-point massage with other treatments such as thermal therapies or electrical stimulation of the muscle.[9]

Warning! Don't Pull Your Leg

Do not, DO NOT use your hands to pull your leg toward your chest. Do not use a belt or a band to pull your leg towards your chest. Use only your own leg muscles to carry out this maneuver and be gentle with your back. If you must, use your fingertips only, to provide some gentle support and guidance to the leg. I have seen two patients cause disc tears by pulling too hard on a belt looped behind the knee. Both of these patients were well meaning, if slightly Type-A personality people, who pulled too hard trying to stretch out the piriformis and in the process brought on severe, if temporary, back problems. Please, please don't be next! This is one place where my recommendations will sometimes split off from those of others who encourage the use of belts and straps. It is really better if you can use your own efforts at mental control to consciously relax the buttock muscles. Never try to "pull them out" by using your arm strength.

ELECTRICAL STIMULATION IS A USEFUL COMPLEMENT

The primary purpose of the electrical stimulation is to fatigue the muscle into a relaxed state. Although the treatment itself can produce a strong tingling or zinging sensation, afterwards the muscle feels very loose.

STRETCHING SPEEDS RECOVERY

You will probably need to do piriformis stretches two to three times a week forever to keep your buttock muscles properly flexible and prevent a recurrence of sciatic nerve compression. Once a nerve has been irritated or damaged to the point of producing pain, it is much more prone to re-aggravation. The basic piriformis stretches will be demonstrated to you first by your physical therapist, but there are two related stretches that are widely used: the knee-to-chest stretch and the knee-to-opposite-shoulder stretch. You begin both by lying on the back with your pelvis in a neutral position. Flex both knees and place your feet on the floor about shoulder width apart. Now flex your hip on the good side so that the knee moves towards the chest. Your ability to bring the knee up to the chest will depend on your abdominal girth and your overall flexibility. As you are making this movement, don't focus on achieving the maximum flexion, but concentrate your mental energy on relaxing the muscles deep in your buttock. With time, this movement-with-relaxation will become easier.

KNEE-TO-OPPOSITE SHOULDER STRETCH

This begins the same way, with you lying on your back and your feet planted on the floor. This time, as you bend the hip, angle the movement of your knee so that it is directed towards the opposite shoulder. Obviously, you're not going to actually bring the knee up all the way to the shoulder, but angle it across the abdomen and chest as if you are aiming for the opposite shoulder. Again, you should **never** use a belt, strap, or your hands to pull the leg towards you. You may use fingertip pressure to gently guide the leg though this movement. Hold the stretch for as long as 30 seconds, breathing in and out, consciously relaxing the deeper muscles of the buttock and then slowly return the leg to its original position. You should repeat this two to four more times and then stretch the opposite hip.

INJECTIONS OFFER TEMPORARY RELIEF

It has become increasing popular to inject the piriformis muscle with a variety of agents, including local anesthetics, paralyzing agents (Botox), and steroids.[10] Most often, these drugs are injected into the muscle using some kind of imaging technology for guidance. Frequently, fluoroscopic (X-ray) guidance is used, although ultrasound guidance has been described.[11] The challenge is that the muscle directly overlies the sciatic nerve. Injection into the sciatic nerve itself is likely to be painful and may induce lasting damage. These warnings aside, for some people injection therapy is helpful, but the effects are not expected to last longer than a few weeks to months.

SEE A SPECIALIST IF SURGERY IS RECOMMENDED

When your doctor recommends surgery, this usually means that your piriformis syndrome represents either a long-standing problem or there is clear evidence for a structural problem. Make sure you have a clear picture of what surgery is planned, what the expected outcomes are (will I be pain-free after the surgery?) and what the anticipated time-course is for recovery and return to work. There are different surgical approaches to treating sciatic nerve compression by various structures; you will probably want to see someone who specializes in this type of surgery.

Be Aware of Injection Inclinations

When your doctor recommends referral to a pain specialist or wants to do an injection, make sure you have had a fair trial of physical therapy or that you understand why physical therapy will not be performed. The current reimbursements used by most insurers heavily reward procedural-based management of medical problems, so a doctor may get paid several times more money for making an injection than for speaking with you and learning more deeply about your problem. Most doctors are only human, and you should not seethe with resentment at the first mention of injections or procedures. However, be mindful of the financial pressures that exist and recognize that caution is needed to protect against the undue influence of healthcare reimbursements on medical decision making.

Warning! Red Flags and Back Pain

One of the reasons healthcare providers talk about "red flags" in the assessment of back pain is that the red flags can provide clues to some of the more worrisome causes of back pain. Things like cancer and infection are capable of producing nerve compressions, but these types of events are often associated with other symptoms, such as recent fatigue, recent weight loss, the presence of a known cancer elsewhere in the body, recent fevers and chills, and having had a recent bacterial infection (pneumonia, urinary tract infection, etc). All of us who have had medical training have had the experience of finding a cancer or a life-threatening infection in a patient as a cause of back pain. However, these problems remain relatively rare. The detection of problems like cancer and serious infection are part of the reason it is so helpful to have a detailed MRI picture of your back, but it's not always necessary. Be sure to let your doctor, PA, or nurse know if you are having any red flag symptoms (see Chapter 1); it could be the piece of the puzzle that leads to an early life-saving intervention.

Pudendal Neuropathy (Pudendal Neuralgia)

Pudendal neuropathy, or pudendal nerve compression, is very different from sciatic nerve compression in that the usual cause of the compression is not muscle spasm. Pudendal neuropathy can arise from several causes including trauma and extensive bicycle riding.[12] It may be more common in women. The syndrome of pudendal neuropathy can involve buttock pain, but usually it is closer to the midline of the body and extends into the region of the genitals, producing pain, numbness, or sexual dysfunction. In men there may be an association with prostatitis. By comparison, sciatic nerve compression is more commonly felt in the center of the buttock or even in the upper, outer quadrant and then extends down into the leg. Although a relatively benign syndrome of nerve compression due to chronic scarring or fibrosis, pudendal neuralgia can be incredibly painful and disabling. A perplexing and troubling cause of low back/pelvic floor pain, pudendal neuralgia can leave the sufferer in a nearly disabled state as normal activities like sitting, making bowel movements and engaging in sexual intercourse become severely painful. The pain of pudendal neuralgia is often especially miserable for the person experiencing it, and having a pelvic floor problem may be socially isolating.

PUDENDAL NEUROPATHY TREATMENTS
Because pudendal compression is not due to muscle spasm, ordinary physical therapy approaches are less effective; injections, nerve-destroying treatments, or surgery may be used. Sometimes people with pudendal neuropathy pain are managed through the use of a spinal cord stimulator, a thin electrode placed inside the spinal canal to effectively jam the pain signals before they can reach the brain.

Injections for pudendal neuropathy have been performed using local anesthetics, corticosteroids, and other drugs.[13] Injections should only be performed by people who are familiar with the technique and have received advanced training in this area. Make sure to ask: How many they have done in the last year? How were they trained to do this?

Surgery for pudendal neuropathy usually involves the release of a fibrous band deep in the lower buttock. Make sure to discuss with the surgeon, his or her certainty about the diagnosis, the expected outcomes of the surgery (will I be pain free after surgery?) and the anticipated time needed for recovery and a return to daily life (how long will it be until I can drive again?) and the chances that problems will arise.

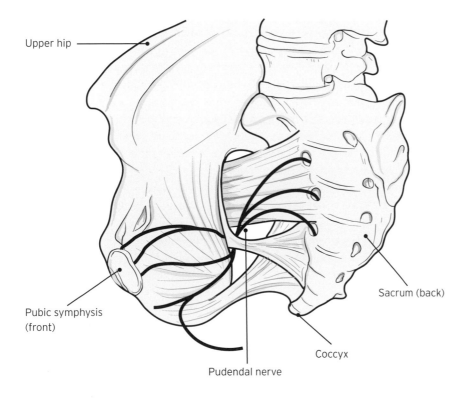

Upper hip

Pubic symphysis
(front)

Pudendal nerve

Coccyx

Sacrum (back)

▲ The course of the pudendal
nerve through the pelvis

What's New: Treatments for Pudendal Neuropathy

- There are descriptions of special tools being used that produce electromagnetic radiation to permanently destroy the nerve.[14] Although this has been described as effective, it sometimes happens that a nerve can grow back after being "destroyed," and when it does, the pain often returns with a vengeance.

- A large study from France recently described the use of ultrasound for the diagnosis of pudendal neuropathy, and reported that this was very helpful in ensuring that the right patients underwent surgery. You can imagine that if you have a surgery to treat a problem you don't actually have, the surgery is not likely to be helpful. For this reason, it's very important to have a solid diagnosis before proceeding to have surgery.[15]

79

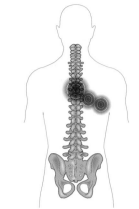

▲ Thoracic nerve root pattern

Other Nerve Conditions That Cause Back Pain

Other conditions may produce nerve pain in the back area. It is important for your doctor to consider other causes of compression if you have nerve pain.

DIABETIC AMYOTROPHY

Diabetes can permanently damage nerves. Many types of neuropathy are associated with diabetes, but one type, called *diabetic amyotrophy*, is thought to be due to sudden nerve damage and is a potential cause of back pain. In this condition, the local blood supply to a nerve may be compromised; what doctors sometimes think of as a mini-stroke in the nerve itself may be the cause of diabetic amyotrophy. In any case, the person with this condition will experience the sudden onset of severe pain in a focused part of the body. Investigations may reveal that the pain is associated with a loss of function of a nerve or nerve root. Diabetic amotrophy can occur in various parts of the body, but when this nerve damage occurs in nerves arising from the thoracic spine or rib area, the pain extends from the back around the rib cage. The pain may be so severe that breathing is limited, a situation that can lead to other problems such as a compromise in oxygen supply to the body or even pneumonia. It is important to note that studies of the complications of diabetes have strongly shown that good diabetic control is critically important to preventing complications such as neuropathy and limiting their severity.

Lyme disease can sometimes produce a syndrome of nerve injury that presents like a mild case of diabetic amyotrophy.

POST-HERPETIC NEURALGIA (PHN)

A distinct cause of nerve-related back pain is post-herpetic neuralgia (PHN). Post-herpetic neuralgia is a chronic pain that first begins with an episode of shingles. Shingles is caused by a reactivation of the chicken pox virus (herpes zoster) in the body. In most people who have been exposed to chicken pox, the virus lies dormant in the body, in part due to suppressive signals from the body's immune system. In certain circumstances, this suppression breaks down and the virus begins to grow and can do so explosively. The results are that the nerve cells that harbor the virus may be damaged or destroyed. The cells most likely to host this takeover by the herpes virus are the sensory nerve cells, often a nerve cell that supplies the skin of the thorax, although the face and other parts of the body can be threatened by shingles. Typically, this occurs in a single nerve root, for reasons that are unknown. Shingles more often occurs in persons who are around 60 years of age, so it is thought that certain age-related changes in the immune system raise the likelihood of shingles occurring. Also, stress is noted in some people who develop shingles, leading to the idea that severe emotional stress can sometimes disable part of the immune system's ability to suppress the virus from reproducing.

If treated immediately, shingles may not progress to the chronic and deeply painful condition of PHN. The characteristics of early shingles is an unusual tingling that progresses the next day to pain in a very focused region (a single dermatome or nerve root distribution). A bumpy rash may or may not be obvious at this stage, but if present, the rash should be focused on the same area as the pain. You should contact your doctor immediately if you suspect shingles. If you cannot see your doctor, PA, or nurse that same day, consider seeking urgent care through another route because if the shingles converts to PHN, it is then devastatingly painful for months and sometimes even years.

VERTEBRAL FRACTURE

Another important potential cause of nerve compression pain is vertebral fracture, this is discussed in some detail in Chapter 8. When vertebral compression fracture involves nerves in the thorax, it can produce a very difficult syndrome of nerve pain that wraps around the body and makes breathing difficult.

NERVE COMPRESSION AFFECTING THE FOOT AND LOWER LEG

Other nerve compression syndromes are not associated with back pain. For example, tarsal tunnel syndrome involves compression of the tibial nerve supplying the front part of the foot (almost like carpal tunnel, but in the foot) and peroneal nerve compression syndrome (more recently called the *fibular nerve*) occurs outside the knee. There are also compression syndromes of the nerves to the front of the leg (the femoral nerve and its branches), such as meralgia paresthetica, a painful compression of the nerve supplying the skin on the outside of the thigh, as well as compression syndromes affecting nerves that supply the front of the groin and the lower abdomen. These are also not typically associated with back pain and should probably be evaluated by a neurologist or other specialist.

What Your Doctor Needs to Know

Your doctor needs to know if you are having the following symptoms in association with your nerve pain: weight loss, fevers or chills, severe pain at night, pain that is worse with lying down, weakness, loss of control over urine or incontinence of bowel or bladder, or numbness over the genital area. Your doctor needs to know what medicines you've been taking, including all over-the-counter medications, as well as what you can and cannot do because of your back pain.

Testing For Nerve Compression

Testing for nerve compression is usually carried out with nerve conduction studies. This is certainly true for the most common nerve compression syndromes: carpal tunnel and ulnar nerve entrapment. These syndromes are most often associated with arm, forearm, and hand pain, although in exceptional situations, some neck pain may be experienced. I occasionally will have a patient tell me that carpal tunnel syndrome produces pain that runs all the way down one side of the body. I don't have a great explanation for this phenomenon except to say that all pain rises to the level of consciousness by passing through several way stations in the spine and brain. In some of these areas, arm and body signals might mix and create false impressions of where the problem actually lies.

There are limits to using nerve conduction tests for the detection of sciatic and pudendal neuropathies. These nerves are located pretty deep in the body, and the surface electrodes used to drive the electrical shocks used for the studies don't penetrate that deeply. As a consequence, other approaches have been adopted. For sciatic nerve compression, a skilled examiner will be able to detect nerve or muscle tenderness deep in the buttock. It is sometimes possible to have a special type of MRI, called MR neurography, performed. In these studies, the MRI signal is optimized to detect the high fat content of the nerve, and 3-D reconstructions are used to detect nerve abnormalities with greater sensitivity. In the case of the pudendal nerve, it may be possible to use a specialized form of ultrasound to detect blood flow through a nearby artery; increased pressure in that artery has been associated with pudendal neuropathy.[16]

The Explanation

The spinal cord is enclosed in the spine, which provides essential protection to spinal nerve roots that travel from spinal cord outward, exiting through spaces between adjacent vertebral bones. Once the nerves exit the spine, they are cloaked in a sheath of fat cells that offer some cushioning, but very little protection from blunt or sharp trauma. This leaves nerves vulnerable to damage from repetitive motions, swollen or fibrotic tendons and ligaments, or in the case of piriformis syndrome, muscles in spasm.

PREVENT NERVE COMPRESSION WITH GOOD POSTURE AND STRETCHING

Although sciatica due to piriformis syndrome often first arises after some trauma such as a car accident or skiing mishap, the predisposition to sciatic problems is amplified by our computer-focused lifestyle that demands that many of us spend hours sitting in front of computers. The sciatic nerve, although well-padded deep in the buttock, is not really designed for sitting on. It is important that you plan active breaks into every work hour. Make sure to get up, move around, and stretch a little. Stretching the piriformis muscles is something that shouldn't just happen when you're recovering from any injury. If your physical therapist has shown you the knee-to-chest exercises, stick with the program. Make sure your hamstring muscles are properly stretched each day and don't forget your gastroc and soleus stretches. Keeping the weight-bearing leg muscles in proper balance is essential to minimizing your risk for sciatica. Consider adding some wall slides to your routine; your physical therapist can show you how. Keep stretching every week. Make sure to maintain a proper body mass and get in plenty of walking as well as other forms of exercise. Avoid lifting objects that are heavier than you can safely manage and always lift with proper technique. Strictly avoid lifting off to the side and never sit at your workstation with an asymmetrical posture to prevent sciatica and sciatic nerve strain.

CHAPTER RESOURCES

1. Konstantinou, K. and K.M. Dunn. 2008. Sciatica: Review of epidemiological studies and prevalence estimates. *Spine* 33 (22): 2464-2472.

2. Filler, A.G., et al. 2005. Sciatica of nondisc origin and piriformis syndrome: Diagnosis by magnetic resonance neurography and interventional magnetic resonance imaging with outcome study of resulting treatment. *J Neurosurg Spine* 2 (2): 99-115.

3. Tiel, R.L. 2008. Piriformis and related entrapment syndromes: Myth and Fallacy. *Neurosurg Clin N Am* 19 (4): 623-7.

4. Nevin Lam, A.C., S.S. Singh, and N.A. Leyland. 2008. Catamenial sciatica. *J Obstet Gynaecol Can* 30 (7): 555, 556.

5. Mollo, M., E. Bautrant, A.K. Rossi-Seignert, S. Collet, R. Boyer, and D. Thiers-Bautrant. 2009. Evaluation of diagnostic accuracy of Colour Duplex Scanning, compared to electroneuromyography, diagnostic score and surgical outcomes, in Pudendal Neuralgia by entrapment: A prospective study on 96 patients. *Pain* 142 (1-2): 159-63.

6. Meknas, K., J. Kartus, J.I. Letto, M. Flaten, and O. Johansen. 2009. A 5-year prospective study of non-surgical treatment of retro-trochanteric pain. *Knee Surg Sports Traumatol Arthrosc* 17 (8): 996-1002.

7. Travell, J. and D. Simons. *Travell & Simons' Myofascial Pain and Dysfunction: The Trigger Point Manual, 2nd edition*. Baltimore: Lippincott Williams & Wilkins, 1998.

8. Davies, Clair. *The Trigger Point Therapy Workbook*. Oakland, CA: New Harbinger Publications, 2001.

9. Shah, J.P., J.V. Danoff, M.J. Desai, S. Parikh, L.Y. Nakamura, T.M. Phillips, and L.H. Gerber. 2008. Biochemicals associated with pain and inflammation are elevated in sites near to and remote from active myofascial trigger points. *Arch Phys Med Rehabil*. 89 (1): 16-23.

10. Kirschner, J.S., P.M. Foye, and J.L. Cole. 2009. Piriformis syndrome, diagnosis and treatment. *Muscle Nerve* 40 (1): 10-8.

11. Smith, J., M.F. Hurdle, A.J. Locketz, and S.J. Wisniewski. 2006. Ultrasound-guided piriformis injection: Technique description and verification. *Arch Phys Med Rehabil* 87 (12): 1664-7.

12. Leibovitch, I. and Y. Mor. 2005. The vicious cycling: bicycling related urogenital disorders. *Eur Urol*. 47 (3): 277-8.

13. Fanucci, E., G. Manenti, A. Ursone, N. Fusco, I. Mylonakou, S. D'Urso, and G. Simonetti. 2009. Role of interventional radiology in pudendal neuralgia: A description of techniques and review of the literature. *Radiol Med* 114 (3): 425-36.

14. Rhame, E.E., K.A. Levey, and C.G. Gharibo. 2009. Successful treatment of refractory pudendal neuralgia with pulsed radiofrequency. *Pain Physician* 12 (3): 633-8.

15. Mollo, M., E. Bautrant, A.K. Rossi-Seignert, S. Collet, R. Boyer, and D. Thiers-Bautrant. 2009. Evaluation of diagnostic accuracy of Colour Duplex Scanning, compared to electroneuromyography, diagnostic score and surgical outcomes, in Pudendal Neuralgia by entrapment: A prospective study on 96 patients. *Pain* 142 (1-2): 159-63.

16. Ibid.

17. Konstantinou, K. and K.M. Dunn. 2008. Sciatica: Review of epidemiological studies and prevalence estimates. *Spine* 33 (22): 2464-2472.

18. Papadopoulos, E.C. and S.N. Khan. 2004. Piriformis syndrome and low back pain: A new classification and review of the literature. *Orthop Clin North Am*. 35:65-71.

19. CDC. "Shingles vaccine," http://www.cdc.gov/vaccines/vpd-vac/shingles/vac-faqs.htm. Accessed January 9, 2010.

Q & A *with Dr. Murinson*

What is piriformis syndrome?

Piriformis syndrome is a condition in which the sciatic nerve is compressed between two muscles as it passes through the deep part of the buttock. The typical scenario leading to this condition is accident-related trauma, whether from a car accident or a fall. The piriformis muscle is involved in connecting the sacrum (base of the spine) to the top of the thigh bone (greater trochanter of the femur) and contributes to our ability to externally rotate the leg. When the piriformis muscle is injured and in spasm, there may be a radiating pain down the leg. Piriformis syndrome can produce pain that is deep, severe, especially bothersome at night, worse with prolonged sitting, and sometime radiating to and beyond the knee. The pain can be felt up into the lower back. This pain will usually not respond to over-the-counter medications and can be fairly resistant to prescription medications as well. If you think that you may have piriformis syndrome, you should seek out qualified medical care. Ask your current doctor, nurse, or PA if they have had any training in physical medicine or rehabilitation medicine. It is important to have skilled guidance as you seek to address this problem.

My doctor tells me piriformis syndrome is rare; how rare is it?

Conservative estimates for the occurrence of piriformis syndrome in those with back pain are as low as five percent, although some have reported estimates as high as 32 percent.[17] Now, if you stop to consider that the lifetime chances of having back pain are 80 percent, then piriformis syndrome might not really be so rare. Imagine a city of 100,000. If 80 percent will have back pain over a lifetime, and five percent of those are due to piriformis syndrome, which means that 4,000 people in that small city will experience piriformis syndrome at some point in their lives. Now multiply that by over 300 million Americans![18]

Should I get the vaccine against shingles?

If you are 60 years or older, the CDC recommends that you get the shingles vaccine. Shingles is the common name for the herpetic rash that leads to PHN (post-herpetic neuralgia). Getting the vaccine will cut your chances of developing PHN by two-thirds and is generally considered safe. There are some people who should not get the vaccine so make sure to check with your doctor and read up on the vaccine in advance.[19]

CHAPTER 5

Sacroiliac (SI) Joint Dysfunction

Diagnosis can be tricky. Be sure to ask questions and get an expert medical opinion.

the DIAGNOSIS

> Do you have pain that is located to one side of the spine?

> Does your pain seem to sit heavily in the base of the back just off to the side? Does it stab sharply with every step or effort to shift your weight?

Pain on one side of the lower back that worsens with every step is usually due to a dislocated sacroiliac (SI) joint. If you can take one finger and locate your maximal pain halfway between the spine and hip in the lower back, you may have SI joint problems. Sometimes, certain movements will temporarily relieve the pain; however, the pain of a dislocated SI joint can be so severe as to make normal walking impossible. The pain of a dislocated or destabilized SI joint may be aching or breathtakingly sharp. Activities such as rising from a chair or stepping off a curb can make this pain worse.

Back pain due to a dysfunctional SI joint needs expert medical assessment and care, but it is important to know that there is some degree of controversy about the best way to diagnose SI joint dysfunction. As no one test is considered definitive, it is often necessary to subject a patient to a series of tests, some of which may provoke pain in the SI joint. At times, an X-ray of the SI joint will be needed. It may be necessary to include other tests as well, because the pain of SI joint dysfunction shares some features with other causes of back pain. Your doctor may order a nerve conduction test to make sure that the problem is not caused by damage to nerves arising from the spine. (This test is described in detail in Chapter 2). Once all the test results are in, a clearer picture will emerge. The possibilities range from "nothing is clearly wrong" to a "clear joint disruption" to "subtle signs of SI joint problems."

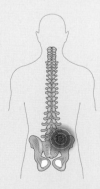

What's New: A Major Pain in the Back

In research studies about the causes of low back pain, a surprising number of people with "low back pain" were found to be suffering from SI joint dysfunction. Estimates of the number of people actually suffering from SI joint dysfunction as a cause of back pain are between 10 and 30 percent. The largest study found that SI joint dysfunction explained the pain of 22 percent of patients with low back pain. Other major causes of back pain include disc problems, such as herniation and disc tears.[1]

CLUES TO DIAGNOSIS

To test for SI joint dysfunction, probe for painful areas on the back. If you can identify a single spot, located two to three inches from the midline of the base of back, where moderate pressure with the fingertip produces an extreme pain response, you may have SI joint dysfunction. Another test is to lie on your back with a partner positioned next to you. Have your partner place his or her palms on the front parts of your hip bones, one hand on either side. Your partner should press downward, applying steady pressure to both sides at the same time. This maneuver is supposed to cause the front side of the SI joints to open and will produce pain in some patients with SI joint dysfunction. If this maneuver worsens your pain, you may need to have SI joint-focused therapy; read on!

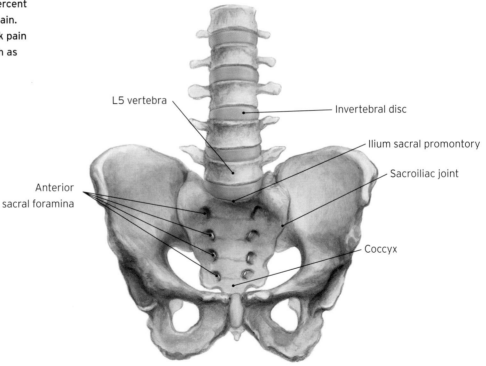

L5 vertebra

Invertebral disc

Ilium sacral promontory

Sacroiliac joint

Anterior sacral foramina

Coccyx

the PRESCRIPTION

If you have a dislocated SI joint:
- Your doctor will very likely recommend physical therapy, especially if there is no perceptible weakness. The effectiveness of SI joint therapy depends on the skillfulness of the physical therapist or chiropractor; the nature of the joint dislocation; and the motivation of the person undergoing treatment to consistently follow exercise recommendations.
- Your doctor may recommend injection of the SI joint with pain-active medications such as lidocaine or cortisone. These medications may provide temporary relief from pain, and may allow the physical therapist a window of opportunity for more aggressive treatments, but injections such as these are not shown to provide a lasting benefit.
- Your doctor may recommend that you wear an SI band or belt. This will depend on whether it seems to be a one-time problem or happens again and again despite the use of other treatments.
  - An SI band is a moderately heavy belt that straps around the hips to provide external pressure on the pelvis
  - The success of SI band therapy depends in part on the wearer's ability to get a comfortable fit and to wear the band when needed.

Painful SI Joints During Pregnancy

The sacroiliac joints are prone to develop painful instability during pregnancy as a result of hormones that loosen the normally tremendous strength of the ligaments. In this loosened state, a certain degree of play in the joint can develop. Under the stresses of walking and carrying additional weight around without respite, these normally silent joints can become very painful. Although the surrounding muscles normally play a minimal role in supporting the joint, when the ligaments are softened, the muscles become more important to joint stabilization. Fortunately, it is possible to provide relief to the overtaxed ligaments and joint structures through muscle strengthening exercises.

(continued)

WHAT IF YOUR DOCTOR DIAGNOSES INFLAMMATION OF THE SI JOINT? In this case, it may be necessary to be tested for medical conditions that predispose to inflammation of the SI joint.

WHAT IF YOUR DOCTOR FINDS THAT YOU HAVE SYMPTOMS OF SI JOINT DYSFUNCTION BUT NO EVIDENCE FOR DISLOCATION ON X-RAY? The SI joint is designed to be resiliently stable, as it is subjected to profound stresses every time weight is transferred from leg to leg. Your imaging studies may not show clear-cut signs of dislocation, but SI joint dysfunction is a diagnosis based on the pattern of pain and the clinical exam results. A trial of SI joint therapy may very worthwhile as the basic skeletal manipulations are usually not harmful and the core muscle strengthening exercises used for the treatment and prevention of SI joint dysfunction are almost always beneficial. In rare cases, pain in the SI joint area is due to a mass (tumor), an infection (abcess) or a fracture. These serious but rare causes of pain in this area are readily assessed through the other diagnostic tests described further in this chapter. The treatment for these conditions is individualized.

The Treatment

If your doctor recommends "physical therapy first," this usually means that you have the type of SI joint dysfunction best treated without surgery (the vast majority of SI joint dysfunction is treated without s urgery). Several treatment modalities fall under the umbrella of physical therapy as the primary treatment for SI joint problems: manual therapies, thermal therapies, electrical stimulation therapies, traction/inversion therapies, and conditioning and strengthening.

MANUAL THERAPIES ARE HIGHLY EFFECTIVE

Manual therapies can reverse and resolve an initial episode of SI joint dysfunction. In fact, anecdotal evidence suggests that the best chance of a cure for SI joint dysfunction may be to obtain an immediate reduction of the joint dislocation by a practitioner skilled in manual therapies. There are several approaches to reducing stress on the SI joint, some of which involve fairly complicated positioning of the legs and body and require significant strength on the part of the person performing the treatment.

One example of a maneuver that can decrease SI joint strain is as follows: Working with a partner, first lie on a table-firm bed with your bad side down. Keeping your bad leg straight, bring the knee of your good leg up towards your chest by flexing the hip and bending the knee, then allow the lower part of your good leg to rotate downward a bit, until your foot is placed in front and rests flat, supporting you from in front. Have a partner grasp the ankle of your bad leg, keeping the knee straight, gently move the foot in a horizontal plane until the hip is flexed at about 25 degrees, and then gently raise the leg in a vertical direction. If anything about this does not feel right or hurts, stop immediately and seek medical assessment. When properly performed, this maneuver can relieve stress on the SI joint and may be used by a manual therapy practitioner such as a physical therapist to reposition the joint that is dysfunctional. In actual practice, the complex nature of the SI joint means that the dysfunction may result from joint malpositioning in one of several directions. For example, in many people, SI joint dysfunction limits the movement of the bones on either side of the joint in a forward and back direction. For others, SI joint dysfunction may mean that the bones of the joint have shifted their relative positions in an up-down direction. Therapy will vary depending on the particulars of the problem.

(Painful SI Joint During Pregnancy continued)

Squeezing a ball between the knees is one example of an exercise that can relieve sacroiliac pain. Gluteal tightening exercises and Kegel exercises are also critical components of exercising for relief of SI joint pain in pregnancy. If these measures—undertaken with medical supervision—fail to resolve the problem, a sacral belt may contribute some external compression to stabilize the joint. For sure, it is very important to wear flat shoes once problems with SI joint pain in pregnancy develop. Heels will increase the amount of force delivered to the body with each step, and throw the body into an alignment that increases the stress on the pelvis.

PHYSICAL AND THERMAL THERAPIES RELAX THE MUSCLES

Physical therapy can include the use of thermal therapies, including warm compresses and cold packs. These therapies can help to control pain and relax the muscles around the joint. The muscles that surround and support the SI joint can both respond to joint pain by going into spasm, worsening the pain, and potentially make the SI joint dysfunction more intractable and resistant to treatment. Thermal therapies are an important part of a comprehensive physical therapy program and are widely acknowledged as medically necessary.

ELECTRICAL STIMULATION THERAPIES ARE WIDELY ACCEPTED

In theory, the continuous electrical stimulation applied via sticky electrodes attached to the skin will cause the muscle to go into an exhausted state that mimics normal relaxation. This offers yet another way to break the pain and spasm cycle that often arises in muscle and impedes normal function and recovery. Although mildly uncomfortable for some, electrical stimulation therapy is a useful complement to other approaches used in physical rehabilitation. It allows the therapist to target specific muscle groups, is generally without side effects, and can spare patients from being exposed to higher doses of oral muscle relaxants.

STRENGTHENING AND CONDITIONING ARE ESSENTIAL

Relatively few muscles actively contribute to holding the SI joint together, so many of the exercises used to treat SI joint dysfunction are actually stretching exercises; others are designed to strengthen nearby core muscles. You will need to consult with a skilled physical therapist, as the exercises during the acute phase will depend on which side the problem lies. More often than not, the SI joint is painful on one side and less so on the other. Although opinions on this vary, it seems there are multiple ways in which the SI joint can become "out of joint." This is evident from the absence of a single definitive test to diagnose SI joint dysfunction and from the variety of repositioning maneuvers that are used to restore normal functioning. Once your physical therapist has provided you with a specific prescription for realigning your SI joint, you will likely need to perform core exercises in the future to prevent recurrence of this problem.[2]

INJECTIONS PROVIDE SHORT-TERM RELIEF

If your doctor recommends treatment with a pain injection, chances are this may provide some immediate relief and help to confirm the diagnosis of SI joint dysfunction as a cause of your pain. Most of the time, injection of the SI joint for pain relief is performed under CT or X-ray guidance (fluoroscopic-guided). In the majority of cases, the injection will consist of a mixture of lidocaine, a numbing agent, and a sustained-release form of cortisone. The lidocaine can act within seconds to provide relief of pain from SI joint dysfunction; however, the effects of lidocaine typically last only a few hours. It is common for pain to return later in the day after an injection has provided initial relief. The cortisone agent is injected because over a period of a few days, it will begin to provide similar pain relief, and in this case, the pain-relief may last for two or more weeks.

In patients who have unbearable pain from SI joint dysfunction, the pain injection may be a necessary intervention. However, research suggests that the long-term effects of these injections are insignificant. It is not expected that the injection will improve the long-term prospects of a patient with SI joint dysfunction unless it is used in concert with other approaches. Repeated injections of pain-active medicines is not practical beyond a few attempts as a risk for infection is always present and the cortisone agent may lead to increases in the infection risk as well as weakening the nearby muscles and bones.

ORAL MEDICATIONS ALLEVIATE SUFFERING

If your doctor recommends that you take pain medications by mouth, chances are this will be just one of the necessary steps to address your SI joint dysfunction. Oral pain medicines, although helpful for alleviating pain and suffering, are unlikely to be successful for treatment if other measures are not taken.

Many medications can be used for the treatment of pain related to SI joint dysfunction. These include over-the-counter medications such as acetaminophen, ibuprofen, and naprosyn. However, some physicians may prefer medications that are available by prescription only for SI joint-related pain. In your physician advises you to take a prescription pain medication, make sure to ask the doctor and your pharmacist about the potential side effects. Discuss any potential concerns before starting the medication, and read over the literature about the medication carefully. If your physician prescribes medication that contains opioids, make sure you have a plan for preventing and treating any constipation. Opioids are known to produce profound and potentially life-threatening constipation. The best strategy is to begin a "bowel regimen" designed to prevent constipation before problems start. Although essential during opioid use, good hydration is unlikely to be enough to ward off problems. More aggressive strategies like drinking prune juice, taking a bulk-forming laxative with lots of hydration, or taking a bowel stimulating agent, such as Senna, are likely to be needed.

Core-Strengthening Exercises

1. Pelvic-neutral abdominal strengthening exercises such as a pelvic tilt, crunches, leg extensions, and a modified bridge position

2. Back crunches, which are described in detail in the muscle pain chapter, but basically involve lying on the stomach and raising both arms and legs from the floor for a count of 30

3. Inner-thigh strengthening, which can be done by lying on the back with a ball between the knees and squeezing the knees together for 15 seconds and relaxing with five to 10 repetitions each day

4. Outer-thigh strengthening, which can be performed using an elastic band around the legs at the knee level while lying on the back in a pelvic-neutral position. Press the knees apart against the resistance of the band for 10 seconds and relax, repeating several times each day.

5. Avoid stretches that place asymmetrical strain on the pelvic structures, like the hurdler's stretch. This may worsen SI joint dysfunction.

Testing for SI Joint Dysfunction

Several different types of bedside tests can be used to determine the nature of a problem suspected to be SI joint dysfunction. The following tests are widely used by experienced clinicians.[3,4]

DISTRACTION TEST

The patient lies on his or her back on the examination table. The examiner places one hand on each of the front facing parts of the hips and presses down toward the table. This pressure is believed to distract or separate the anterior parts of the SI joint away from each other and may produce pain in the joint that is malfunctioning.[5]

COMPRESSION TEST

The patient is asked to lie on his or her side while the examiner applies downward pressure on the up-facing hip.

SACRAL THRUST

The patient is asked to lie on the stomach while the examiner applies downward pressure on the center of the sacrum. A modification of this test is the Yeoman's test, which involves lifting one leg up toward the ceiling while applying pressure over the sacrum.

THIGH THRUST

The patient will lie on his or her back. The examiner will guide the patient to bend one leg up at the hip until the knee is pointing up to the ceiling. Placing one hand under the sacrum for stabilization, the examiner will apply downward pressure to the thigh that is vertically oriented.

PELVIC TORSION TEST (GAENSLEN'S TEST)

The patient is asked to lie on the less painful side facing away from the examiner. The examiner may stabilize the top hip with one hand, and will then pull the upper leg (affected side) backward, extending the hip and putting stress on the SI joint.

FABER'S TEST

FABER is actually an acronym for Flexion, Abduction, and External Rotation. This describes the movements of the hip joint as the test is performed. In this test, the patient is asked to lie on his or her back. The leg is supported by the examiner who bends the hip into flexion, guides the thigh outward to the side (abduction of the hip) and then rotates the calf and foot (clockwise for the right leg) to externally rotate the thigh at the hip joint. This maneuver places strain on the SI joint and may provoke pain when the joint is dysfunctional. This is also called *Patrick's Test*.

SACRAL SULCUS TENDERNESS

Palpation over the area of the SI joint may provoke pain in patients with SI joint dysfunction so that tenderness in this area is supportive of the diagnosis, but not definitive as there are other reasons why a person will have tenderness in this area.[6]

GILLET'S MOVEMENT TEST

While the patient is standing, the examiner places fingers on the back to help identify the relative motion of various structures during the test. The patient is then asked to raise one leg by flexing the hip and knee, bringing the leg forward and up as far as possible without losing balance. In patients with unrestricted movement at the SI joint, the finger located over the bone landmark on the hip will move downward slightly as the SI joint accommodates this change in position.

The Explanation

The back and spine are dynamic musculoskeletal structures that rely on a solid foundation for proper function. The pelvis, a heavy ring of bone lying between the hips, connects the legs to each other and provides foundational support to the spine that is essential for ordinary movements.[7] Certain conditions—especially pregnancy but also accidental trauma—can cause damage to the structures of the pelvis. When the pelvic ring is disturbed, movements that are typically pain-free and seemingly effortless can become impossible to accomplish.

The sacroiliac joints are a pair of large joints connecting the sacrum to the hip bones on either side. Early in life, the surfaces of the bones inside the joint are smooth, but over time the bones develop ridges and valleys. The most prominent of these is a central ridge on the sacrum bone running along the longest dimension of the joint, complemented by a valley in the face of the hip bone where it sits opposite the sacrum. This adaption in form may contribute to the stabilization of the joint. Major contributions to the phenomenal stability of the sacroiliac joint are made by very heavy ligaments that bind the sacrum and hip bones together in the back most strongly, but also in the front (inside the pelvis). This structural arrangement contributes substantial strength but also allows for some flexibility and shock absorption. The ring of the pelvis consists of the two hip bones on either side meeting in the front, as well as the sacrum in back. This means there are a total of three joints to form the pelvic ring: two sacroiliac joints and one joint in the front.

What to Look for with Low Lateral Back Pain

- Pain is much worse when you press on it, in an area two to three inches (5 to 8 cm) lateral to the spine base.[8]

- Weakness may be perceived but this is only when pain is very sharp; what may be more evident is a feeling of instability, lacking a strong base of support, or discombobulation.

- Signs of sacroiliac dysfunction include pain that is worse with standing from a sitting position and pain that is worse when weight is transferred to one leg, in particular when walking or stepping off a curb.

Any of these can become painful but only the two in back are referred to as sacroiliac joints and are associated with back pain. In very elderly people, parts of the sacroiliac joints may fuse. In some cases, there is a focused inflammation of the joint. This is typical of a rheumatological condition called *ankylosing spondylitis*.

The sacroiliac joint is richly innervated with pain-sensing nerve fibers. The nerve fibers that supply the joint arise from 12 or more different nerve roots extending from the 2nd lumbar level to the 3rd sacral level. This may explain why SI joint pain is sometimes difficult to pinpoint and can manifest in many different ways.

CHAPTER RESOURCES

1. Schwarzer, A.C., C.N. Aprill, and N. Bogduk. 1995. The sacroiliac joint in chronic low back pain. *Spine (Phila Pa 1976)* 20 (1): 31-7.

2. Hertling, Darlene and Randolph M. Kessler. *Management of Common Musculoskeletal Disorders: Physical Therapy Principles*. Philadelphia, PA: Lippincott Williams and Wilkins, 2006.

3. Young, S., C. Aprill, and M. Laslett. 2003. Correlation of clinical examination characteristics with three sources of chronic low back pain. *Spine J* 3 (6): 460-65.

4. Petty, Nicola J. *Neuromusculoskeletal Examination and Assessment: A Handbook for Therapists*. Churchill Livingstone, 1997.

5. Laslett, M., et al. 2005. Agreement between diagnoses reached by clinical examination and available reference standards: A prospective study of 216 patients with lumbopelvic pain. *BMC Musculoskelet Disord*. 9 (6): 28.

6. Dreyfuss, P., et al. 2004. Sacroiliac joint pain. *J Am Acad Orthop Surg*. 12 (4): 255-65.

7. Norris, Christopher M. *Back Stability: Integrating Science and Therapy, Second Edition*. Champaign, IL: Human Kinetics, 2008.

8. Fortin, J.D. and F.J. Falco. 1997. The Fortin finger test: An indicator of sacroiliac pain. *Am J Orthop (Belle Mead NJ)* 26 (7): 477-80.

9. Forst, S.L., M.T. Wheeler, J.D. Fortin, and J.A. Vilensky. 2006. The sacroiliac joint: anatomy, physiology and clinical significance. *Pain Physician* 9 (1): 61-7.

10. Goode, A., E.J. Hegedus, P. Sizer, J.M. Brismee, A. Linberg, and C.E. Cook. 2008. Three-dimensional movements of the sacroiliac joint: A systematic review of the literature and assessment of clinical utility. *J Man Manip Ther* 16 (1): 25-38.

Q & A *with Dr. Murinson*

What causes SI joint dysfunction?

Trauma as a result of falls and motor vehicle accidents can lead to SI joint dysfunction. This can include major trauma such as a fall landing on the buttocks, a rear-impact car accident, especially where one foot is stabilized on a pedal, and side-impact motor vehicle accidents. In cases where ligaments are damaged by prior injury or weakened, minor trauma such as stepping especially hard off a curb or bending sideways to lift a heavy grocery basket can be sufficient to initiate an episode of SI joint dysfunction. Conditions that result in asymmetries across the pelvis may increase chronic stresses on the joint and predispose people to SI joint dysfunction; these could include scoliosis, leg-length discrepancies, chronic weakness in one leg, and hip-flexor deconditioning (iliopsoas contracture).[9]

What makes sacroiliac dysfunction distinguishable from other kinds of back problems?

Sacroiliac disease worsens with standing from a sitting position and becomes worse with provocative maneuvers, a series of bedside tests that some physicians will use to confirm the diagnosis of SI joint dysfunction. The joint moves only miniscule amounts under normal circumstances, with one or two millimeters of movement-induced shape change being the typical extent of motion.[10] For this reason, physical therapists and other knowledgeable healthcare providers will ask patients if getting up from a chair provokes pain.

Are any other back problems associated with SI dysfunction?

Several specific medical conditions are associated with inflammation of the sacroiliac joint. Among these, ankylosing spondylitis is a condition in which patients most frequently develop inflammation of the SI joint as part of the syndrome. This inflammation is usually painful and can be diagnosed with an X-ray. Patients with ankylosing spondylitis also experience a collapse of the spine. It is this spinal collapse that produces the characteristic forward curvature of the spine and can eventually lead to difficulties with holding the head upright. Other inflammatory diseases, including reactive arthritis, arthritis of psoriasis, and arthritis associated with inflammatory bowel disease are also known to produce sacroiliac inflammation and pain. The treatments for each of these are tailored to the specific disease.

CHAPTER 6

Facet Disease

Physical therapy is often the best course of action.

> ❯ **Do you have back pain that is focused on one side of the back?**

> ❯ **Does your pain get a lot worse when you try to bend backwards, such as when you look at the sky, or when you make a twisting motion?**

Pain that is much worse with backward bending (extension of the back) is often due to an inflamed or injured facet joint. One way to test for facet joint disease is to begin by standing with your feet firmly planted on the ground and then, maintaining your balance, bend the upper half of your body back as if you are trying to look at a spot on the ceiling while experiencing a stiff neck (try not to tip just your head back). If this worsens your pain, facet joint disease may be the cause.

Facet joint pain can be very focused and intense. At other times, facet joint pain can be part of a larger problem. When a vertebral disc collapses, for example, one or both of the paired facet joints at the same level in the back will experience severe stress. At its most severe, facet joint disease can lead to nerve root compression and pain that radiates into the leg. The bottom line is, if your back pain is interfering with your ability to twist around and to bend backwards, you may have facet disease; read on!

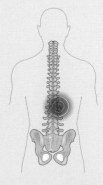

the PRESCRIPTION

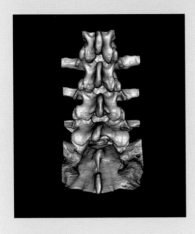

▲ Facet joins

▼ Pain when bending backwards

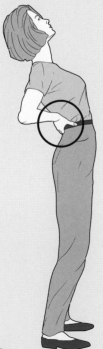

Back pain due to facet disease needs expert medical assessment and care. Sometimes an X-ray, MRI, or CT scan will be used as a first diagnostic test. Some doctors may be familiar with specific bedside tests to check for facet joint problems, while others may not. In cases where the pain in your back extends down into the leg and it's not clear what the cause of the pain is, your doctor may order a nerve conduction test as part of the evaluation for your pain. Some doctors, and some clinical trials, will only make a definitive diagnosis of facet joint pain after showing that the pain is relieved by a numbing injection into the joint, but in many cases this is not required to proceed with treatment.

If you have facet joint pain (sometimes referred to as *Z-joint pain*):

- Your doctor will likely recommend physical therapy, especially if this is the first time you're having this pain and the pain is problematic but not unbearable. For those who prefer to avoid potential problems with medications and needle-based approaches to treatment, physical therapy is often the best course of action.
- Your doctor may recommend an injection into the joint, especially if the pain is severe and if your doctor is familiar with these techniques. The facet joint injection is typically performed under fluoroscopic (X-ray) guidance, so there may be limitations to using this approach in all patients.

WHAT IF YOUR DOCTOR DIAGNOSES AN INFLAMED FACET JOINT?

Because facet joints are like most other joints of the body, they can become inflamed (or infected) much like the knee, wrist, or other joints of the body can. In these cases, it may be most effective to begin therapy with the injection of a drug into the joint space. In many cases, the injected drugs will include a quick-acting numbing agent; this will allow you and the doctor to know that the right spot has been injected. Most times, the injection will also include a longer-acting, steroid-based medication. The steroid will serve two purposes; it can reduce inflammation and will also tend to decrease the amount of pain.

WHAT IF YOUR DOCTOR DIAGNOSES A FACET DISLOCATION?

Facet joint dislocation is rare in the lumbar spine.[1] More commonly occurring in the neck, facet joint dislocation is typically the result of some trauma and is detected by X-ray, CT, or MRI. If an actual facet joint dislocation is identified, the treatment will vary depending on the location and severity of the condition. In the neck, approaches to treatment range from stabilization with a soft collar and immobilization with a "halo" or hard collar to surgery and neck fusion. Facet joint dislocations in the mid-back or lower back should be managed by someone with medical expertise in this area.

WHAT IF YOUR DOCTOR FINDS THAT THE FACET JOINTS ARE DEGENERATED AND NERVES ARE BEING PINCHED?

In some cases, especially when facet joint disease is severe and associated with vertebral fracture, bony malformations, or collapsed vertebra or disc, surgical management of the facet joint disease may be considered. If a facet joint is severely degenerated, it may develop bony spurs that protrude into the spaces that normally exist between adjacent vertebral bones. When this happens, the exiting nerve roots can be compressed and pain can radiate into the leg. In advanced cases, weakness can accompany the nerve root compression and surgery will be favored as a best choice. In some cases of severe disease, physical therapy may still be beneficial. Make sure to discuss the treatment options with your healthcare provider.

Warning! A Window of Pain

One limitation of injections that combine a numbing agent with a longer-acting steroid is that the numbing agent typically wears off before the steroid agent has any noticeable effect on pain. The usual experience is that a person will feel relief for a few hours after an injection, only to have the pain return later that night. The pain-relieving effects of the steroid may not be perceivable until a couple of days have passed, and sometimes longer.

The Treatment

In almost all situations where facet joint disease is the cause of back pain, physical therapy will be an important part of the treatment program. Several components contribute to a comprehensive physical therapy regimen for facet joint pain: thermal therapies, electrical stimulation therapies, manual therapies, traction/inversion therapies, and conditioning and strengthening. In addition, injections may be used to manage pain or confirm the diagnosis, and in rare cases, surgery may be an option.

THERMAL THERAPIES ARE FIRST-LINE TREATMENTS

Typically used at the start of physical therapy, thermal therapies are often continued because they are very effective at getting control over mild-to-moderate pain associated with facet joint disease. In most cases, warm thermal treatments are soothing, can help improve the pliability of muscle, and increase blood flow. At the same time, cold thermal treatments can block pain signaling and potentially short-circuit inflammatory responses to injury and vigorous activity.

CYST IN FACET JOINT

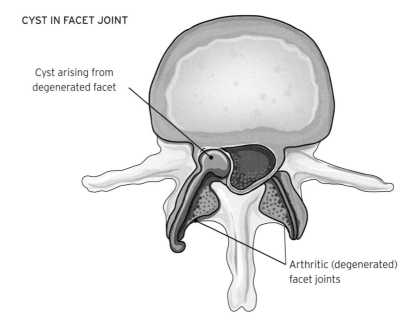

Cyst arising from degenerated facet

Arthritic (degenerated) facet joints

ELECTRICAL STIMULATION RELAXES THE MUSCLES

Electrical stimulation therapies are one of several approaches that may be used to get specific muscles in the back to relax. Because the body often responds to pain by tensing various nearby muscles, abnormal muscle contractions do occur in association with facet joint pain. In the case of facet joint pain, these contractions not only contribute to the overall intensification of pain, but may actually perpetuate the problem!

MANUAL THERAPIES CAN PROVIDE LASTING RELIEF

Manual therapies for facet disease include trigger point massage and mobilization of the spine. Trigger point massage is a specialized technique of using focused pressure on specific locations in the muscle to induce relaxation. This is not the same as feeling more relaxed; it is an actual physiological response of the muscle that can be measured with electrical probes, often palpable to the person performing the therapy, and is sometimes visible to the eye as a barely perceptible twitch. Regardless, the accomplished practitioner of trigger point massage can produce lasting relief and change the course of therapy for the better.

TRACTION AND INVERSION THERAPIES REDUCE PRESSURE

As we age, the discs in the back gradually lose not only resilience but height. The collapse of disc height means that the facet joints must change with the upper surface of the joint sliding downward over the face of the lower surface. There is a lot of play in the covering of the joint so that this shift does not usually strain the joint capsule, but the mechanics of the joint do change in the process, and cartilage of the joint may be stressed or eroded as a consequence. Gentle traction or inversion can help reduce some of this strain.

STRENGTHENING AND CONDITIONING

These therapies are so important to treating and preventing facet joint disease that this chapter should probably begin and end with back-strengthening exercise. Because of the construction of the spine only as a stack of bones would not be sufficient to support a lifetime of running, walking, lifting, sitting, etc., the muscles must be viewed as an integral part of the spine. It is the part of the spine that you have the greatest direct control over. Exercises for facet joint disease should begin with core strengthening, with the back in a supported position.

Begin with the pelvic tilt exercise, described in Chapter 5. Wall slides are a great exercise to strengthen core muscles while supporting the back so that facet joints won't hurt. To do a wall slide, stand with your back to a wall, about 15 inches (38 cm) from the wall. Place your feet shoulder width apart and pointing

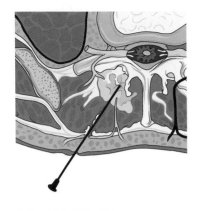

▲ Facet joint injection

forward. Use your hands to guide you back until you're leaning against the wall, then slide your bottom down a bit as if you were going to sit in a chair. Make sure your knees are over your feet and hold this position for a few seconds. Increase the time that you hold this position until you can remain there for 30 seconds comfortably, then move your feet a little further out and try to slide further down. Work on going gradually lower with your wall slides until you are comfortable "sitting" against the wall for 45 seconds. Be careful not to overdo it with this exercise, as it can flare up any knee problems. Back extension exercises, done gently at first because the pain of the facet is made worse by extension, are critically important to long-term management of facet joint pain. The classic back extension exercise is described in Chapter 1. Other key exercises include core muscle exercises such as described in Chapter 14.

INJECTIONS CAN CONFIRM THE DIAGNOSIS

If your doctor recommends a facet joint injection right away, make sure that this seems like the best choice for you. Many doctors will use facet joint injections to definitively establish the diagnosis of facet joint pain. The injection typically includes a combination of medicines designed to immediately numb the joint (a local anesthetic) and reduce any inflammation in the joint (a steroid). These medicines are injected as a mixture through a single needle. Be sure to let your doctor know if you might be allergic to drugs in either of these classes of medication. The facet joint injection is typically done with fluoroscopic (X-ray) guidance and should be performed by someone who is very familiar with this procedure.

SURGERY TO MANAGE SEVERE CASES

If your doctor indicates that surgery is the best treatment option, make sure that you have a clear picture of what's wrong with your back and what the planned surgery entails. There are times when surgeons will recommend surgery for management of facet joint problems that are especially severe. Possibilities might include surgery to relieve potential pressure points on nearby nerves, removal of part of the bony covering of the spine and even fusion of the spine in certain circumstances. You will probably want to consult with two or more surgeons before proceeding to surgery for the treatment of facet joint problems. Ask the surgeon what their expectations are for your recovery from surgery. Do they expect that this surgery will relieve the pain completely, mostly, or partially? Will you still need to take pain medicine? How likely is the surgery to improve your quality of life? What are the chances for problems down the road?

Testing for Facet Disease

One problem with bedside testing for facet joint disease is that, as simple as the techniques are, very few "regular" medical doctors will have had sufficient training in this area to be able to perform the studies in a short office visit.[2] In order to obtain a clear diagnosis of facet joint disease, you may need to seek the opinion of an expert in pain medicine, rehabilitation, or physical therapy. If you think that facet joint disease is part of your back problem, you may need to prompt your doctor to think of this diagnosis and possibly refer you for an expert assessment.

One test for locating facet joint disease is to have a person lie down on their stomach. The examiner will then apply pressure with the finger tips over each of the facet joints in turn. This test requires some experience in order to know how much pressure to safely apply to the spine. An examiner who is too ginger will not uncover the problem effectively, and one who is to forceful will produce unnecessary suffering. It is not recommended to try this at home.

The Explanation

The bones of the spinal column are connected to each other through a series of joints. The most familiar of these is the joint at the disc (discussed in detail in Chapters 2 and 3), but there are also two important joints at the back of each vertebra called *facet joints*.[3] The facet joints are paired, one on either side of the spinal canal. They are almond- to ovoid-shaped connections between vertebral bones that add support and flexibility to the spine. Compared to the joint at the disc, the facet joints are more like the other joints of the body in construction and are prone to some of the same problems that other joints suffer: arthritis, dislocation, inflammation, degeneration, and even infection. The facet joints are located at each of the spinal levels. The location of the pain associated with a particular facet joint often follows a characteristic pattern.

The facet joints are designed to provide both stability and flexibility to the spinal column. Oriented in a vertical direction between the vertebrae at the base of the spine, the facet joints allow movement forward and back (bending over and arching back). The facet joints in the thoracic spine are angled and in this part of the spine, movement is relatively restricted due to the presence of the ribs and rib cage. In the neck, the facet joints are more horizontally oriented, an arrangement that permits the turning movement of the head. In the low back, facet joints are aligned vertically, allowing for bending forward and back.

In many cases, the facet joint is damaged by years of chronic use and abuse. As the vertebral discs dry out and flatten with age, additional stress is placed on the facet joints. There is a fair amount of "slack" in the covering of the joint in early life, which allows the two sides of the joint to glide past each other when

Warning! Beware of Nerve Block Procedures

In some cases of facet joint disease, the pain specialist may propose a nerve block procedure. In extreme cases, some doctors will recommend destruction or ablation of the nerve believed to be carrying the pain signals. If someone suggests this type of procedure to you, make sure not only that you understand the immediate risks (and benefits) of the procedure, but also that you are told, in clear terms, how likely it is to provide pain relief six months or a year later. Many times, nerve ablation is a temporary fix to a long-lasting problem. Despite appearing to be an ideal solution, it's not practical to just cut the nerve to a painful part, even a little part like the facet joint. This is almost never effective for two reasons: 1) severe pain seems to induce lasting changes in the nervous system so that even if the nerve is cut, a persistent pain signal may already be embedded in the system, and 2) the nerve almost always tries to grow back. It's been observed clinically that even when cutting the nerve fixes the problem at first, most people will experience a return of the problem over the months that follow, and many times the problem is even worse than it was initially.

What's in a Name?

The facet joint is more properly known by its anatomical name, the *zygapophyseal joint* (try saying that three times fast!). It is also known in shorthand as the *Z-joint*.

bending and twisting motions occur. When the vertebral disc flattens down, however, the two sides of the joint assume new—more or less permanent—positions relative to each other, placing a chronic strain on the joint. The bones of the joint will often respond to chronic strain by a process of overgrowth called *osteophyte formation*. Osteophyte formation is a process whereby the edges and corners of bones will heap up and develop protrusions and bony spurs. These areas of overgrowth can intrude into the spaces usually occupied by nerves, and when this happens, nerve pain can result.

Another consequence of chronic facet joint strain is degeneration of the cartilage in the joint. When this happens, you essentially have arthritis in the back. Like any joint with arthritis, the facet joint can be persistently inflamed and achingly painful. The typical measures for treating this are described in this chapter but include stretching, strengthening, mild traction, the use of anti-inflammatory medicines, and even ice. More extreme measures can include nerve injections, nerve destroying procedures, and in rare cases, spinal fusion.

CHAPTER RESOURCES

1. Cox, J.E. and W.J. Vanarthos. 1995. Unilateral dislocation of the lumbosacral facet joint: Imaging features. *Journal Emergency Radiology* 2 (4): 234-6.

2. Young, S., C. Aprill, and M. Laslett. 2003. Correlation of clinical examination characteristics with three sources of chronic low back pain. *Spine J* 3 (6): 460-5.

3. Giles, Lynton and Kevin Singer. *Clinical Anatomy and Management of Low Back Pain*. Butterworth-Heinemann, 1997.

4. Bogduk, Nikolai. *Clinical Anatomy of the Lumbar Spine and Sacrum*. New York: Elsevier, 1987.

5. Dreyfuss, P., C. Tibiletti, and S. Dreyer. 1994. Thoracic zygapophyseal joint pain patterns. *Spine* 19 (7): 807-11.

What is a *pars defect* and how does it relate to facet disease?

The pars is part of the posterior ring of each vertebra, linking the superior and inferior facet joint faces. The full name of the pars is the *pars interarticularis* (loosely translating as "the part between the joint faces"). A *pars defect* is a deficiency in the pars, due either to a failure of the bone to form properly after birth or a fracture. The pars defect disconnects the posterior part of the vertebral ring from the anterior part of the vertebra.

The pars defect relates to facet disease due to the interlinking aspects of the spine's construction: each vertebra is stabilized from in front and in back. In order for a facet joint to become dislocated or serious damaged, either the disc will have to shift or the bones will have to give, which they do by fracturing. A pars defect can be present from birth as part of a minor spinal malformation. Alternatively, a pars defect can be a fracture of the vertebral ring. These fractures can result from a specific accident or trauma, but can also occur when excessive force is applied to the spine through heavy lifting.[4] A pars defect may either be of minimal significance or require management by a surgical specialist, depending of the location and extent of the problem.

What does facet joint pain feel like?

Facet joint pain can occur in either the lower, middle, or upper back, or even in the neck.[5] It is usually most intense off to one side of the spine, and the level of the pain is usually near but not necessarily limited to the specific level of the problem. The pain of facet joint disease is usually due to arthritis or inflammation, so sensations of dull aching, strong pain, and even sharp twinges are not atypical. Facet joint pain is different from the pain of a back muscle problem, in that it lasts for much longer periods of time and is especially brought on by extending the back. Activities such as painting ceilings, changing light bulbs in suspended fixtures, or trimming trees are likely to provoke pain in people with facet joint disease.

CHAPTER 7

Spinal Instability

(Spondylolisthesis)

OTC medications, heating pads, exercise, and corsets to stabilize the spine are often the best remedy for pain.

the *DIAGNOSIS*

> Do you have pain that is very severe at times and at other times is almost nothing?

> Does your pain seem to flare up in discrete episodes and settle down, only to flare up again?

> During an episode, do you have difficulty standing upright and develop muscle tightness especially in the hamstrings?

Pain that is severe at times and comes and goes in discrete episodes can be due to spinal instability. In this condition, simple movements such as standing up from a low toilet may be enough to trigger a shift of the vertebral bones relative to one another. Sometimes, the bones shift into a position that is more properly aligned; when this happens, pain is relieved. At other times, one vertebral bone will shift forward or back relative to the one below it. When the two vertebral bones are not lined up properly, this is called a *spondylolisthesis* (spon-di-lo-lis-thee-sis). The ligaments, disc, and joints are all stressed, and incapacitating, severe pain may result.

The syndrome of spondylolisthesis is especially characterized by tight hamstring muscles. One way to check if your hamstrings are tight is to do a straight leg raise test. When you lie on your back and have a helper lift one of your legs gradually up in the air, bending only at the hip, your hamstrings are tight if there is tightness or pain in the back of your thigh that limits the range of upward movement in your leg. (Pain in the back with this movement is more indicative of a nerve root compression from a disc.) Have the helper check the other leg with you as well.

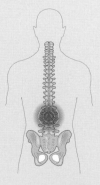

Rare Causes of Spinal Instability

In rare cases, spinal instability is due to a mass (tumor), an infection (abscess), or a spinal malformation. These problems are readily assessed through MRI and the other diagnostic tests described here. The treatment for these conditions is individualized.

Another characteristic of spondylolisthesis is that the pain in the back worsens as the spine is extended, as when someone bends backwards to look up at the ceiling. This is because spondylolisthesis is most typically associated with damage to the boney arch portion of the vertebra, and this part is pressurized with backwards bending of the spine.

If you have lived with the experience of "having your back go out" repeatedly and the cause is not a bulging disc or muscle spasm, you may have spinal instability; read on!

DISPLACED VERTEBRA CAUSING PRESSURE ON NERVE

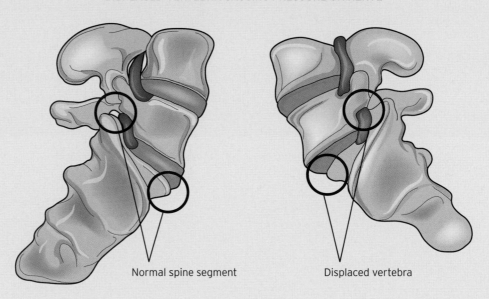

Normal spine segment   Displaced vertebra

the PRESCRIPTION

Back pain due to spondylolisthesis needs expert medical assessment and care. If you have a spondylolisthesis (sometimes referred to as a *spinal instability* or a *spinal misalignment*):

- Your doctor may recommend over-the-counter pain medication and conservative measures such as a heating pad, especially if the spinal misalignment is believed to be old and not related to your pain.
- Your doctor may recommend physical therapy, especially if the misalignment is mild and there is no evidence of nerve compression. Surgery may still be needed if non-surgical treatments are ineffective and if the misalignment appears to be worsening over time.
- Chiropractic therapy may be appropriate for some forms of spondylolisthesis. Sometimes more than one treatment visit is needed.
- Non-surgical decompression therapy may be beneficial, but solid evidence in support of this new approach is still accumulating.
- A corset can be used to help stabilize the spine and relieve pain.
- Your doctor may refer you to a surgeon, especially if there is nerve-related weakness, persistent disabling instability, or advanced spinal degeneration. Surgery has advantages and disadvantages; however, if there is obvious weakness or loss of control over bowel or bladder, emergency surgery may be necessary to preserve function.

A Corset, Of Course

You may be advised to wear a corset, and this may help to reduce movement around a hypermobile spine segment. You might wonder if the corset is a permanent state of affairs, but with proper rehabilitation and careful self-awareness, it is possible for the muscles to gain strength and support the spine, for the ligaments to repair somewhat, and for the pain-amplification cycle to wind-down.

WHAT IF YOUR DOCTOR DIAGNOSES A PULLED MUSCLE?

A pulled muscle will usually improve in three to five days. The difference between a pulled muscle and a spondylolisthesis is that spondylolisthesis attacks occur again and again, always with the same type of pain. Usually, the pain is deeper and sharper than the typical burning quality of muscle pain.

WHAT IF YOUR DOCTOR DIAGNOSES A BULGING DISC?

In this case, physical therapy and exercise are usually best. The degree of pain and disability associated with this type of injury varies greatly, but in this case you can do a lot to improve your chances of a fast and full recovery.

WHAT IF YOUR DOCTOR FINDS THAT A NERVE ROOT IS BEING COMPRESSED BY AN OVERGROWTH OF BONES (BONY SPURS) OR LIGAMENTS IN THE LOWER BACK?

The overgrowth of bones and ligaments in the lower back is usually the end result of years of accumulated trauma to the back. It carries the label of degenerative joint disease (DJD). Surgery may be an alternative, but this depends on the extent of damage to the spine. Many times, physical therapy and programmed exercise is the right solution.

The Treatment

If your doctor recommends physical therapy first, this usually means you have a mild spondylolisthesis or one that is prone to reduction with mild-to-moderate levels of pressure or traction. The types of physical therapy treatments used for spondylolisthesis are similar to those used for injured discs (see Chapter 3). Treatment for spondylolisthesis may emphasize manual therapy and traction approaches in order to restore the normal alignment of the vertebral bones.[1] If you want to avoid surgery now or in the future, you will need to do your recommended back-strengthening exercises every day. Some of the exercises that are useful for strengthening the spine and preventing shifting into and out of spondylolisthesis are described in Chapter 14. But make sure you check with your doctor or physical therapist before proceeding.

A GOOD EXERCISE FROM PILATES

One exercise that is good for building stronger spine muscles comes from Pilates. Begin by lying on your back; make sure to hold a solid pelvic neutral position at the start and throughout. Straighten one leg and bend the knee of the other, placing the foot on the floor firmly. Now, extend the arms fully as if you are lifting them over your head (see below). Raise the heel of the straight leg about four inches (10 cm) off the floor, then flex the knee and hip, bringing the knee up toward the chest. As you do this, bring both arms over you in an arc that aims to place one arm on either side of the flexed leg. As you do this, you should slightly bend your upper body up in a modified abdominal crunch. Return the arms and the flexed leg to their extended position and repeat this movement five to 10 times. Then switch legs and readjust the arc of your arms to exercise the other side of the body.

COSTLY COMPUTER-CONTROLLED THERAPY

If your doctor recommends decompression therapy, be aware that many insurance companies are not going to pay this therapy. In the past, Medicare has not paid for this, so it is essential that you check with your medical insurer before making a decision, as it can cost thousands of dollars. There are different forms of this device; however, one machine is designed to apply controlled traction on the spine while simultaneously delivering electrical stimulation to the back. The idea is that if the electrical stimulation can relax the back and block muscle spasms, the traction will be more effective. Many patients have reported a benefit from this therapy, but the ordinary standards for proving that the therapy works have not yet been met.

SPINAL ADJUSTMENTS BY A CHIROPRACTOR

If your doctor recommends manual therapy or spinal manipulation, make sure that you feel comfortable with the treatment plan. Many insurance companies will pay for spinal adjustments and chiropractic care. Ask whether the treatment is expected to work in one or a few visits, or whether protracted therapy is anticipated. Spinal adjustments to the lumbar spine are generally safe and effective.

In terms of caring for the lower back, chiropractors often have a distinct advantage over the garden-variety M.D. in the extent of training that they receive in disorders of the back and spine. Chiropractor training is essentially focused on the spine and how disorders of the spine impact the overall health of the body.[2] The well-prepared chiropractor will have received a much more detailed theoretical understanding of spine mechanics and greater working knowledge of effective mechanical solutions to spine problems through their training. The chiropractor will usually approach a back problem with a can-do, hands-on attitude and will excel in doctor-patient communication. In general, chiropractors do not prescribe medications, as this is counter to the philosophy that they are trained in, and they do not perform surgeries. The number of chiropractors in the U.S. is still small, compared with the number of physicians and surgeons, but these numbers are expected to grow, according to the Bureau of Labor Statistics.

Warning!

There have been documented cases of major strokes to the brain occurring at five times the baseline rate in adults younger than 45 years of age following chiropractic treatments.[3] It has been proposed that this is especially associated with high-force chiropractic manipulation of the neck.[4] The reason the strokes are believed to occur is because the blood vessels that supply the back half of the brain are threaded through small holes on the sides of the neck vertebral bones (like a thread running through beads on a string). The explanation that seems to follow is that as the high-force manipulation causes the neck vertebral bones to twist and slide against each other, the blood vessels can be exposed to shearing forces and become blocked as the vessel is compressed or damaged.

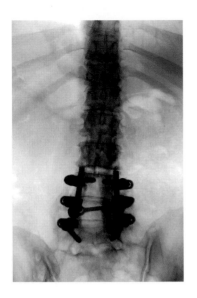

▲ X-ray of the lumbar spine with a spinal fusion

Checklist for the First Visit to the Surgeon (Before the Surgery):

○ Copies of imaging studies

○ List of questions for surgeon

○ Brief summary of the problem

○ List of other medical conditions

○ List of medications

○ Pain calendar

○ Support person

Surgery Means Spinal Fusion

If your doctor refers you to a surgeon right away, chances are that you have a spinal instability that is putting your spinal cord or nerve roots at risk without surgical intervention. The surgical procedures that may be used to address a spondylolisthesis include spinal fusion. Other surgical procedures may be considered as appropriate by the surgeon. Spinal fusion is a major procedure. It's a process of fusing or permanently linking different vertebral bones together into one unit. Fusion can involve fusing two adjacent vertebrae together with bone from elsewhere, sometimes harvested from the patient's own hip (bone autograft). At other times, another source of bone is preferred; if the bone comes from someone else, it is referred to as an *allograft*. The usual source of bone for allografts is deceased donors; you will hear this called the *bone bank*. Spinal fusion can also entail the placement of metal rods and screws alongside and into the spine. Fusions that use metal rods and screws are sometimes called *fusion with instrumentation*. The use of metal rods allows for the spine to be stabilized over multiple spinal segments at once, and can be used to stabilize a bone fusion until it is solidly fused. A brief description of the actual procedure follows.

NUTS AND BOLTS OF SPINAL FUSION

Spinal fusion is an established surgical procedure that usually requires a long incision on the back. Although some surgeons are adopting a new type of fusion surgery that is done through surgical keyholes in the abdomen, most spinal fusions continue to be performed using a long-incision-over-the-back approach. Once the incision has been made, the surgeon will separate the layers of fat, muscle, and connective tissues that are attached to the bone, which will anchor the fusion hardware. Holes are drilled into the bone that forms the sides of the boney arch on the back part of the target vertebrae. These holes may be tested to make sure that they are stable and can hold a screw. The screws are designed to connect to plates or rods that will fix the vertebrae in place. Oftentimes, screws and plates are used together with grafted bone in a fusion surgery, as these metal structures will prevent shifting as the bone solidifies and hardens. The maturation of the fusing bone takes several weeks. Once the plates or rods are in place, the screws can be tightened and locked into place. The surgeon will then close the incision in the back, cleansing the incision and working to control any bleeding as needed. A dressing will be placed in the operating room and this dressing will remain in place until the surgeon determines it should be removed.

PREPARATION FOR SURGERY

Before seeing the surgeon, there are some things you should do to prepare: gather your relevant medical records, make a list of potential questions, and make sure you have a support person who will stay with you throughout the visit. Make sure that you have the necessary imaging studies, both reports and films. If blood work or other tests have been performed, bring copies of those reports as well. Have an accurate list of your medications including dietary supplements, and take a list of your prior surgeries. Make sure to alert the surgeon and staff to prior problems with anesthesia, bleeding, or procedures.

Consider taking a notebook or an audio recording device to the visit as information can flow very quickly once treatment decisions are made. Always ask permission before making an audio recording of your visit. If the surgeon is recommending surgery, make sure you know what procedure is planned, whether the procedure might change based on findings at the time of surgery, and what the anticipated course of recovery might be. Have a reasonable sense of the expected limitations on activity after surgery. If you are planning airplane travel, make sure to get specific guidelines. If you smoke, you must quit before spinal fusion surgery. The biggest risk factor for failed fusions is smoking; it is believed that the nicotine kills bone cells.

After your first surgical office visit, read over the materials that you receive. Make sure you understand what procedure is planned, how many days you will stay in the hospital, whether a rehab center stay is expected, and how much time off from work will be needed. Make sure you feel comfortable with the plan. You will need to know how to prepare for the surgery, including when to stop NSAIDs (potentially contributing to excess blood-thinning) and how long to fast before the surgery. Ask if you will need to complete a pre-operative exam and determine if any exercise is recommended or restricted beforehand.

The day of surgery, you will be meeting someone from the anesthesiology team before the surgery begins. Make sure that they know how long you've been fasting, what medications you normally take and have taken in the last 24 hours, and how long you have been off NSAIDs (including aspirin, ibuprofen, naprosyn, etc.).

POST-SURGICAL CONSIDERATIONS

After surgery, you will have some degree of pain. Most of the time, post-surgical pain is controlled with strong pain medication. Opioids are widely used during and after spine surgery. If you have been on pain medications before the surgery, you may need to make sure the pain team is aware of this and makes any necessary adjustments.

Chiropractic Interventions Gain Support

The research in support of chiropractic interventions is building. Studies suggest that chiropractic care is beneficial, but these studies are small and usually focus on chronic low back pain generally rather than any specific diagnosis.[5] Studies also indicate that chiropractic care is effective at relieving pain and disability, associated with high levels of patient satisfaction, and less expensive than primary care management of back pain.[6]

What's New: Smoking Puts Fusion at Risk

A recent study on spinal fusion indicated that smoking doubles that chance of fusion failure. Just 10 cigarettes a day were enough to put people into the higher risk category for fusion failure. Those who quit smoking reduced their risk to fusion failure to near-normal levels.[7]

Good: neutral spine

Bad: Increased curve

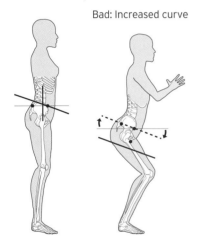

▲ Proper standing posture

Details on what to expect after surgery are covered in Chapter 2, but make sure you follow recommendations on when to get out of bed, when to ask for assistance, and how to move around in the first few days. You will need to have rehab after spinal fusion surgery. Be careful not to overdo it, because the spinal fusion takes several weeks to become strong against the ordinary pressures placed on the spine.

Take the pain medication that is recommended, but be sure to communicate with your nurses and doctors if you think the pain is more than you expected. Out of the ordinary pain after surgery can be a sign that something is amiss; don't suffer in silence. In addition, too much pain can interfere with the normal recovery process. The body will release stress hormones in response to pain and this will block healing. People with excess pain are prone to falls, you definitely don't want to risk falling at this stage!

You should not smoke after spinal fusion surgery. Make sure to eat a diet that is varied and high in fiber. Stay well hydrated and act aggressively to prevent any constipation while on opioids (sometimes call narcotics) such as Percocet, oxycodone, or codeine.

Testing For Spinal Instability

Many times, a basic X-ray of the back is the best test for the diagnosis of a spondylolisthesis.[8] However, it is possible that the X-ray may not reflect the problem if it is taken at a time when the alignment has self-corrected. If the spine is very unstable, it may be helpful to have flexion-extension X-rays, where the pictures of the spine are taken as the person bends forward and back. An MRI may or may not be helpful. If you have pain that is shooting down the leg, especially pain that extends below the knee, or if you have actual weakness along with pain, your doctor may recommend a nerve conduction test to assess whether the nerves in the back are still intact. This test is described in detail in Chapter 2. Once imaging and other test results are in, a clearer picture will emerge. The possibilities range from "nothing is wrong" to a "mild misalignment" to "high-grade misalignment of the spine."

A spondylolisthesis is described by specialists using two systems. The first is a system that tries to identify the causes or origins of the problem. This diagnostic classification system includes labels such as dysplastic (meaning improperly formed during development), isthmic (pertaining to the boney arch structure), traumatic, and degenerative. The other descriptive system is based on the degree of slippage that has occurred between the involved vertebral bones. In this system, a grade is assigned. A Grade I slippage is less than 25 percent displaced, a Grade II is 25–50 percent displaced, and so on. The higher the grade, the more likely the spondylolisthesis is to compress nerve roots and other structures. It is asserted in the medical literature that low-grade misalignment that is stably displaced is not necessarily painful. A low grade slippage that moves in and out of alignment is more likely to be painful.

The Explanation

The vertebral bones of the spinal cord are stacked one on top of the other like blocks in a child's tower. Most of the time, extraordinarily strong ligaments in the back hold these bones in proper alignment, but in some cases, if the spine has been injured or stressed, one of these bones may begin to shift in and out of alignment. The most common scenario is that the vertebral bone that sits on top will slide forward (an anterolisthesis). The less common scenario is that the vertebral

Warning! Using NSAIDs May Interfere with Bone Healing after Surgery

Medical literature suggests that NSAIDs may interfere with bone healing, and laboratory-based research is quoted as supporting this. Recently, the recommendation was made that surgeons should not only avoid the use of NSAIDs immediately before and after surgery, but that they should counsel patients to discontinue NSAID use well in advance of the surgery.

It is important to note that most surgeons will require NSAIDs be stopped for a specific period of time prior to surgery because of the risk of blood-thinning effects.[9]

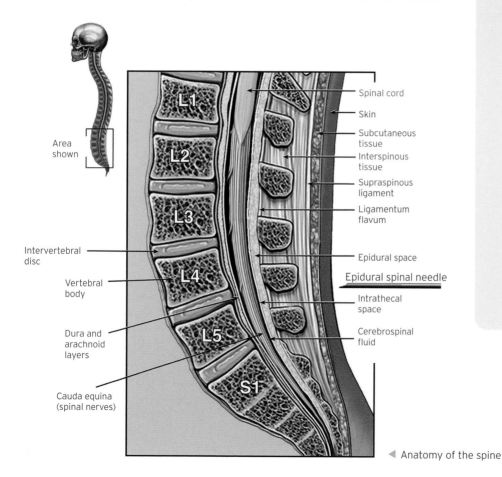

Area shown

L1
L2
L3
L4
L5
S1

Spinal cord
Skin
Subcutaneous tissue
Interspinous tissue
Supraspinous ligament
Ligamentum flavum
Epidural space
Epidural spinal needle
Intrathecal space
Cerebrospinal fluid

Intervertebral disc
Vertebral body
Dura and arachnoid layers
Cauda equina (spinal nerves)

◀ Anatomy of the spine

117

The Pros and Cons of Spine Surgery

If you are contemplating spinal fusion surgery for treatment of spondylolisthesis, don't expect miracles. The spine fusion is intended to immobilize part of the spine. You will need to exercise care in returning to daily life. There is a good body of evidence that shows that the spine above and below the level of the fusion is subject to increased stresses. For people who don't adapt well to life after spine fusion, it can almost seem like there is a pattern of spreading spine degeneration. Increased body awareness can be helpful if it does not make you so fearful of doing anything that your world begins to contract. Stay focused on positive health but as you do, include a plan to care for your back in your overall health picture.

bone on top will slide back (a retrolisthesis). Although that are some misalignments that are thought to be relatively stable, others will be meta-stable and will slip in and out of alignment. For these people, this slippage can sometimes be accompanied by excruciating pain and difficulty getting into a fully upright posture.

It is widely believed that having an exaggerated low back curvature (lordosis) or sway back posture with the buttocks protruding increases the chance of spondylolisthesis occurring. This is because the L5 vertebral body sits on a sloping angle and this slope is exaggerated when the low back curvature is increased. This is an important reminder to keep a constant watch on the spine and work on maintaining a pelvic neutral position even when standing. One way to facilitate this is to think about tightening your buttocks and curving your tail bone under as you stand. Another helpful visualization is to think about pulling your belly button toward your spine.

CHAPTER RESOURCES

1. McNeely, M.L., G. Torrance, and D.J. Magee. 2003. A systematic review of physiotherapy for spondylolysis and spondylolisthesis. *Man Ther* 8 (2): 80-91.

2. Bureau of Labor Statistics, U.S. Department of Labor, "Chiropractors," *Occupational Outlook Handbook, 2010-11 Edition*. http://www.bls.gov/oco/ocos071.htm. Accessed 12/24/2009.

3. Rothwell, D.M., S.J. Bondy, and J.I. Williams. 2001. Chiropractic manipulation and stroke: A population-based case-control study. *Stroke* 32:1054-1060.

4. Chiroweb Editorial Staff. Stroke after chiropractic neck manipulation A 'small but significant risk,' says American Heart Association. http://www.chiroweb.com/mpacms/dc/article.php?id=41126. Accessed 12/27/09.

5. Wilkey, A., M. Gregory, D. Byfield, and P.W. McCarthy. 2008. A comparison between chiropractic management and pain clinic management for chronic low-back pain in a national health service outpatient clinic. *J Altern Complement Med* 14 (5): 465-73.

6. Grieves, B., J.M. Menke, and K.J. Pursel. 2009. Cost minimization analysis of low back pain claims data for chiropractic vs medicine in a managed care organization. *J Manipulative Physiol Ther* 32 (9): 734-9.

7. Andersen, T., F.B. Christensen, M. Laursen, K. Høy, E.S. Hansen, and C. Bünger. 2001. Smoking as a predictor of negative outcome in lumbar spinal fusion. *Spine (Phila Pa 1976)* 26 (23): 2623-8.

8. Irani, Z. and J.J. Patel. "Spondylolisthesis," eMedicine. http://emedicine.medscape.com/article/396016-overview. Accessed 12/20/2009.

9. Thaller, J., M. Walker, A.J. Kline, and D.G. Anderson. 2005. The effect of nonsteroidal anti-inflammatory agents on spinal fusion. *Orthopedics* 28 (3): 299-303.

10. Lowe, W. March 2006. Spondylolisthesis: An elusive cause of low back pain. *Massage Today*, 6 (3). http://www.massagetoday.com/mpacms/mt/article.php?id=13380. Accessed 12/30/2009.

11. Towers, S.S. and W.B. Pratt. 1990. Spondylolysis and associated spondylolisthesis in Eskimo and Athabascan populations. *Clin Orthop Relat Res* 250:171-175.

What are the triggers for episodic spondylolisthesis?

The usual scenario for a person with episodic spondylolisthesis is that he or she will have had an episode of strong back pain that resolved before anything was done about it. He or she will do well for a period of time, and then all of a sudden the back pain will return. The things that trigger the episode may seem relatively minor but include getting up from a low toilet seat, bending over into the trunk of a car, playing weekend sports too vigorously, or even sneezing.

If you have episodic spondylolisthesis, you will need to become a keen student of your own body mechanics.[10] You may need to scrupulously avoid activities that put your back out. You may need to avoid low seating, get a special adapter for low toilet seats in your home, and give up on shoveling snow and moving furniture!

Besides those with sway backs, who is likely to get a spondylolisthesis?

Certain activities and sports increase the occurrence of a spondylolisthesis. Populations as special risk include gymnasts, rowers, weightlifter, divers, and football players. Certain professional groups are at increased risk, including loggers and those who carry very heavy packs such as foot soldiers. One group that has consistently been identified as having higher occurrence of spondylolisthesis is the Eskimos. There is some indication that a genetic component may contribute to this.[11] Overall, it is thought that a spondylolisthesis is present in less than 5 percent of the population, although the degenerative form increases with advancing age. An L4-L5 spondylolisthesis is more characteristic of an early-in-life problem, whereas L5-S1 slippage is typical of later-in-life degenerative spondylolisthesis.

CHAPTER 8

Vertebral Fracture: Emergency!

Self-treatment can result in permanent disability. Get emergency medical help as soon as possible.

> **Have you been told by a doctor that you have a fractured vertebra?**

Warning! Do Not Self-Diagnose a Vertebral Fracture

Most of the chapters in this book are written as a guide to learning how to better understand what may be going on with your back. This chapter is different: it is intended as a guide for those who have been told by a physician that they have experienced vertebral fracture. You should not try to self-diagnose vertebral fracture. It is a critically serious medical problem that can result in permanent disability if one wrong move is made. If you suspect that you have a vertebral fracture, stop reading and call 911.

A vertebral fracture can cause the spine to be unstable. Seemingly simple movements, such as trying to sit up, can cause the bones to shift abnormally, crushing the spine or severing blood vessels. Vertebral fracture is often preceded by some trauma, such as a motor vehicle accident, a fall down stairs, or a swimming/diving accident, but in older adults with osteoporosis, the trauma that causes vertebral fracture may be less obvious. If you have osteoporosis or a collapsing spine, the sudden onset of strong pain in the center of the back may be your only sign that serious damage has occurred to the back.

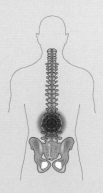

the PRESCRIPTION

Suspected vertebral fracture is a medical emergency for the reason that some types of fracture can result in compression of the spinal cord or injury to other nearby structures. Emergency personnel are trained in how to move people minimizing the of risk for provoking further damage to the body in the event that there is a spinal instability due to a fracture. They will need to methodically evacuate someone with a suspected spine injury, typically using an immobilization board. At the hospital, someone skilled in assessing the spine for fracture will determine if it is "safe to move" by obtaining a medical history (sometimes very abbreviated), doing a physical exam, and evaluating any necessary X-rays or images. The treatments will vary with the severity of the fracture and the degree of associated spinal instability.

If you have a fractured vertebra in the neck:
- Your doctor will have determined the particular characteristics of your fracture on the basis of X-rays and potentially other imaging studies (CT, MRI).
- Your neck may need to be immobilized or surgically fused.
- It may seem that fusion is a drastic solution given that it results in reduced movement in the neck permanently, but if you can still move your arms and legs, that is something to be grateful for. Cervical spine fracture is potentially fatal.

If you have a fractured vertebra in the middle of the back (thoracic region):
- Your doctor will have determined the particular characteristics of your fracture on the basis of X-rays; sometimes other imaging will be needed.
- You may need to take medication for pain.
- Your doctor will discuss with you any procedures that may help stabilize the broken vertebra.
- Make sure you understand if your spinal cord is in any danger of compression.
- Make sure you know the warning signs of spinal cord compression and when to see urgent medical care. (See Chapter 9 for more on spinal cord compression.)

If you have a fractured vertebra in the lower back (lumbar region and sacrum):

- Your doctor will have determined the particular characteristics of your fracture on the basis of X-rays and potentially other imaging.
- If the spine is unstable, your doctor may recommend surgery to stabilize it. Depending on the situation, spinal fusion may be required to stabilize a fractured vertebra.
- Sometimes a brace or corset is used to stabilize the spine if this is considered sufficient to promote healing.
- You may need to take medication for pain.
- You may be instructed to eliminate certain activities for several weeks after fracture. It takes a long time for bones to heal after a break, possibly six weeks or longer. Make sure you know how much activity is permitted during this time and follow your doctor's directions very carefully. Failure to observe activity restriction can result in persistent pain and a worsening of the spinal stability.

Warning! If You Suspect a Vertebral Fracture, Do Not Move!

Vertebral facture is a medical emergency that may result immediately in permanent paralysis or other serious harm. If you ever suspect that a vertebra has just fractured, **do not move.** Have someone call 911 and let the emergency medical team know that you may have spine injury.

If You Smoke, Quit Immediately

If you smoke cigarettes and you've experienced a vertebral fracture, you must quit immediately. Smoking interferes with the body's ability to deliver oxygen to bones and recuperation from vertebral fracture.

What's New: Controversy over Vertebroplasty Efficacy

Major controversy erupted with the publication of two articles in the *New England Journal of Medicine* describing studies of the technique for the relief of back pain and reporting that no benefit was proven.[5] The lead doctor on one study expressed shock with the study's conclusions, as have others.[6] It has been the experience of many physicians that vertebroplasty is very helpful when a patient is experiencing severe back pain from vertebral fracture. In all fairness, it seems that the larger of the two studies showed that there was improvement in clinically meaningful pain relief at one month. Acceptance of this result was limited however, because the result had borderline statistical significance. The patients who received both the actual vertebroplasty and those who received the sham treatment were both better immediately after the procedure. This may reflect the effects of sedation, local anesthetic, or the normal stress response in someone undergoing a medical procedure. For reasons that aren't clear from the published works, neither of the studies was able to recruit the full quota of

(continued)

The Treatment

The treatment of vertebral fracture depends of the location and extent of the fracture. Your doctors will assess the stability of the spine and treatments will include pain control measures and any necessary steps to prevent shifting or collapse of the spinal column.

USE ICE PACKS FREQUENTLY FOR DAYS OR WEEKS

Vertebral fracture will often require ice packs to be used several times daily, for a week or longer. In other parts of this book, ice packs are strongly recommended for the first 48 hours after a minor injury or pain flare, situations of muscle pain, minor insult, or acute back pain. With vertebral fracture, however, ice is often recommended for the duration of the first week, and warm compresses are avoided during this time.[1] This is because in vertebral fracture there is a longer time window for swelling and inflammation that may ultimately interfere with healing. Ice will help reduce both pain and excessive inflammation. Make sure to wrap your icepack in a cloth before applying it, and leave it in place for no more than 20 minutes at a time.

PRESCRIPTION-STRENGTH MEDICINE WILL ALLEVIATE PAIN

When your doctor recommends medication, it is entirely possible that prescription-strength pain medications will be proposed. There is some evidence to suggest that the NSAIDs (non-steroidal anti-inflammatory drugs) can interfere with bone healing, and some orthopedic surgeons avoid NSAIDs after bone surgery. Although a certain percentage of people with vertebral fracture will experience relatively modest pain levels, bones are painful when fractured and a vertebral fracture can result in nerve compression (also painful). For these reasons, it is sometimes necessary to use prescription-strength pain medications, and even still, it is observed that these may not always work for the pain of vertebral fracture. As long as the fracture is healing, you can expect an eventual reduction in back pain.

PHYSICAL THERAPY IS OKAY IF THE SPINE IS ALIGNED AND STABLE

When your doctor recommends physical therapy, this is usually because the integrity and alignment of the spine has not been compromised. Because the spine is an interdependent structure where bones and muscles depend on each other for support and strength, core strengthening is an essential long-term goal for addressing the problems that are associated with vertebral fracture. In the short run, physical therapy can address factors such as pain control, reflex muscle spasm, correcting and reinforcing proper body mechanics in the wake of vertebral fracture, and preventing deconditioning during the acute pain phase.

Physical therapists know exactly how to use ice packs for optimal results; they will position you with bolsters and pillows to place the spine in a rest position and have huge ice packs that they apply over a towel. They will set a timer so that the requisite time is not exceeded, dim the lights, and encourage you to relax for the treatment. It is a good idea to follow this model with ice treatments at home. As you are getting better from your fracture, the physical therapist will show you a series of stretches and exercises. It is absolutely essential to follow through with these. Improving strength and stability of the spine is the single best protection against chronic problems after a spine fracture.

VERTEBROPLASTY STABILIZES THE SPINE WITH GLUE

When your doctor recommends vertebroplasty, you will want to consider this recommendation carefully. Originally devised in the early 1980s in France, vertebroplasty is a procedure in which specialized glue is injected into the fractured vertebra to stabilize and perhaps partially restore the normal vertebral configuration.[2,3] It is considered a minimally invasive procedure that is performed with the patient awake or very mildly sedated with medications to relieve anxiety. A needle is inserted into the fractured vertebra using light X-ray (fluoroscopy) to provide guidance and confirm correct placement of the needle tip. The glue is prepared on the spot in the procedural room because it hardens quickly, changing from something like the texture of toothpaste to a harder-than-bone state in less than 15 minutes. Vertebroplasty has been used for many years and has been believed to be a very successful treatment for severe pain after vertebral fracture. Widely considered a safe procedure, the major limitations were the cost factor and the fact that the technique had never been definitely proven to be effective.[4]

(Whats New? continued)

patients originally planned by the researchers. The Society for Interventional Radiology has weighed in with a Commentary that highlights the limitations of the study and demonstrated pretty effectively that just one additional patient could have swayed the conclusions of the U.S.-based study in the direction of definitely endorsing the treatment. Interestingly, many more sham treatment patients elected to have a second procedure in hopes of pain relief than did vertebroplasty patients.[7]

A CORSET SUPPORTS AND STABILIZES THE SPINE

When your doctor recommends a brace or corset, this usually means that the spine may be mildly unstable but is considered sufficiently stable that a corset will serve to support and prevent abnormal motion of the spine during the healing process. It is especially important to follow your doctor's instructions about activity restrictions very carefully. Wear the corset as instructed, as the purpose of the corset is to prevent motions in the spine that will impede or reverse healing of the bones and ligaments of the spine. It is expect that the corset will aid in relieving pain. This is because if the spine is even mildly unstable and the bones are shifting small amounts, for some people, this is very painful. There are rich supplies of pain-sensing nerve fibers that go to all the structures of the back (except the interior of the vertebral discs). Persistent movements, even when small, can inflame these nerve endings and result in serious pain. A chronic state of mild spinal instability may take the form of intermittent spondylolisthesis (see Chapter 7 for more about spondylolisthesis).

The illustration here shows a type of brace that might be used for spinal immobilization after a vertebral fracture of the mid or low back. This brace is called a *cruciform anterior spinal hyperextension*, or *CASH brace*. It stabilizes the spine in a more upright position and prevents forward bending, which may place further pressure on the vertebra and impede healing.[8] Another type of brace used for this purpose is the Jewett brace.

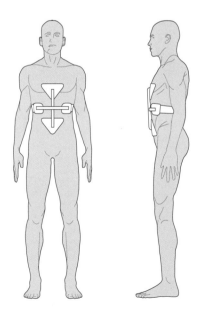

◀ One type of brace used for treatment of vertebral fracture

126

SURGERY IS NEEDED IF THE SPINE MIGHT COLLAPSE

When your doctor recommends surgery, this usually means that a determination has been made that your spine is unstable and that without surgery you are at risk for having the spine shift or collapse and crush part of the spine or some nerve roots. Surgery for vertebral fracture may involve spinal fusion to stabilize the spine. Spinal fusion is described in detail in Chapter 7. In certain cases, it is necessary for special hardware to be placed in the spine to replace or stabilize a seriously damaged vertebral bone. This is done at the time of spinal fusion and is part of that surgery. Your surgeon will discuss this with you if it becomes necessary. You should read the sections on the preparation for surgery, the surgery itself, and the post-surgical considerations in that chapter.

Testing For Vertebral Fracture

Testing for vertebral fracture will usually occur in an emergency room setting, at least initially. Your doctors will want to obtain and review X-rays of the back. CT scans can be very useful for visualizing the bones of the back in more detail, and 3-D renderings are sometimes used. An MRI may be ordered to evaluate the relative location of structures such as nerves, muscles, joint capsules, and ligaments. If someone has been in an accident and placed on an immobilization board at the accident scene, he or she may have to wait for imaging studies for the spine to be "cleared," and then he or she will be unstrapped from the board.

The Explanation

Vertebral fracture is distressingly common. Car accidents, including head-on collisions, vehicular roll-over accidents, and accidents involving impact with windshield and steering wheel are associated with spinal injury.[9] Two main groups of people suffer from vertebral fracture: young adults (mostly male) and older adults who have osteoporosis. In the young adult population, vertebral fracture usually results from serious trauma. Vertebral fracture is associated with spinal cord injury and sadly, there are still 11,000 spinal cord injuries reported each year.[10] Most of these are due to motor vehicle accidents, but violent injury and injuries related to sports such as downhill skiing, diving, and football are important causes of spinal cord injury as well.

Speak Up If You're in Pain

You don't need to suffer in silence. If back pain after vertebral fracture is keeping you awake at night, interfering with your ability to function during the day, or just generally making you miserable, talk with your doctor about treatment options. If that doctor has run out of ideas for pain control, get another opinion. Undertreatment of spine pain is not an acceptable outcome.

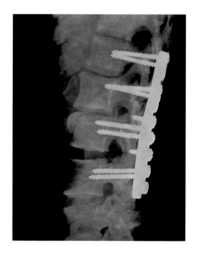

▲ X-ray of a spine showing the metal screws and plates used in the fixation of fractured spinal vertebrae.

Red Flags for People with Vertebral Fracture

The following warning signs, for people who have previously been told they have vertebral fracture by a qualified physician, could indicate that the spinal cord or nerve roots are being compressed or damaged.

- Loss of sensation over the genitals

- Loss of control over urine or feces (incontinence), especially if this is a new problem

- Having difficulty starting a stream of urine as a new problem after back injury

- New severe pain in the back

- Pain or numbness wrapping around the body or leg

- Recent fever or noticeable weight loss

When the spinal cord is injured, communications from the brain to other parts of the body are slowed or stopped. And this is the real danger of vertebral fracture: When a vertebral bone is broken, it can break in such a way that the spinal column becomes unstable; bones can shift or move and wind up pressing on the spinal cord itself, compressing nerve roots or even damaging nearby blood vessels. If you have had a vertebral fracture, a doctor will need to determine your risks for this kind of problem. The consequences of spinal cord injury are potentially severe. A cord injury in the neck can paralyze the hands, arms, and legs, and even stop a person from breathing. These sorts of injuries are potentially fatal when medical care is not provided immediately. When vertebral fracture damages the spinal cord lower down in the back, it may result in leg paralysis and loss of control over the bowels and bladder. These sorts of injuries can leave someone permanently confined to a wheelchair and dramatically shorten the life expectancy. For these reasons, vertebral fracture is considered a medical emergency that requires immediate medical evaluation.

CLASSIFICATION OF VERTEBRAL FRACTURES

Vertebral fractures are classified based on the mechanism of injury and extent of damage. The major classes of injury mechanism include flexion-compression (as in landing in a seated position from a height), axial-compression (as in landing with pressure transmitted straight onto the spine), flexion-distraction (as in the injury produced by a lap belt–only restraint as the spine flexes forward with deceleration), rotational (occurs with extreme side-bending or twisting motions), and shear injuries (where twisting and front-to-back motions are combined). The doctor's evaluation will focus on determining the type of injury, and also whether the various parts of the spine are affected by the injury. In situations of vertebral fracture, attention is focused on three vertical columns, one defined by the front part of all the vertebral bones; one that runs through the middle of all the vertebral bones, top to bottom; and one that runs through the back edge of each of the vertebral bones.

With this information in hand, it will be possible to determine whether the spine is stable, somewhat unstable, or dangerously unstable. The back edge of the spinal bones is bounded by a very strong, fibrous ligament that adds tremendously to the integrity of the whole. If the posterior part of the vertebral bone is damaged and or detached from the ligament, this makes it more likely that the vertebral fracture will be an unstable one. In the illustration, the front column is shaded in blue, the middle column in yellow, and the posterior column in red. The vertebral fracture can disrupt one, two, or all three of these columns. Fractures that disrupt only the front column and some fractures that disrupt the front and middle columns at the same time are still considered stable.

Some examples of how the fracture classification method is applied can be seen in the next illustration. Vertebral burst fractures occur as a result of strong pressure applied directly to the top or bottom of the spine. In the topmost fracture, the front, middle, and back columns of the vertebral bone are all disrupted. This is an unstable fracture. In the middle fracture, the anterior and middle columns are disrupted while the posterior column remains intact. This fracture may be stable. In the bottom fracture, only the middle column is disrupted, and this fracture should be stable. An anterior wedge fracture is the most common fracture associated with osteoporosis. It is most often a stable fracture, but professional evaluation is necessary to make this determination.

OSTEOPOROSIS AND CANCER PRESENT HIGH-RISKS

There are some people who can expect to face significant challenges after vertebral fracture. Two groups in particular are at risk for serious long-term consequences: those with osteoporosis and those who have had a vertebral fracture because cancer is present in the spine. These two situations require different approaches.

For people with osteoporosis, it is important to adopt a program designed to address problems with bone density and bone frailty. If you are not already taking bone-strengthening dietary supplements, this may be your signal to start. Discuss osteoporosis with your doctor. Find out what tests you need done to assess the severity of your osteoporosis and to determine how intensive your treatment for osteoporosis should be. The American Association of Orthopedic Surgeons recommends a DEXA scan as the best test to assess bone density. If you have already had a vertebral fracture but you don't know if you have osteoporosis, you should probably talk to your doctor about getting this very accurate test. There is only a very small amount of radiation involved in the test, about the same that you would receive from so-called background radiation just by living in the United States for three days! There are other tests that are used for screening that are not as accurate and won't provide that much information about what to expect about your risk for future vertebral fractures. At a minimum, every adult needs at least 1000 mg of calcium daily and vitamin D. (See Chapter 21 for more details.)

Osteoporosis is usually seen in people over the age of 50, and certain people are at increased risk. If you are female, tall, slender, and have had minimal weight-bearing exercise throughout your life, you may be at particular risk for osteoporosis. The NIH reports that as many as half of older women may have osteoporosis. People who have been treated with long-term corticosteroids such as prednisone have an even higher risk for osteoporosis. Although steroids can be life-saving in situations such as asthma and autoimmune disease, it is the long-term effects on bone (and skin and muscle) that really limit the benefits of steroids for chronic use.

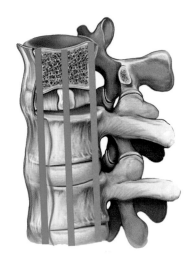

▲ Vertebral fractures are classified by mechanism and by disruption of three vertical columns

THREE TYPES OF SPINAL "BURST"

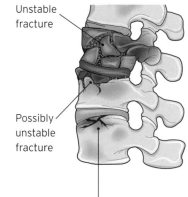

Unstable fracture

Possibly unstable fracture

Middle column fracture, likely to be stable

129

If you or someone you love is living with cancer and has had a vertebral fracture because cancer has weakened the spine, serious measures may be needed to stabilize the spine. Particular cancers, including breast, prostate, and lung, will spread to the bones of the spine. Be aware that pain can be an important symptom of serious problems, and attend to new pain problems carefully. Make sure your doctor knows if there is new or persistent pain in the spine. There are many treatments for cancer in the spine, and you should expect that any pain due to this problem will be taken seriously and a solid action plan put into place. Treatment options can include medications, radiation, and surgery, alone or in combination.

Sometimes vertebral collapse or fracture is due to an infection on the spine. In years past, tuberculosis was seen to invade the spine; this is very rare now as tuberculosis has been effectively treated and reduced in the U.S. Other infections of the bone, such as osteomyelitis, can cause vertebral collapse, and for this reason, fever is considered a warning sign in concert with sudden-onset strong back pain.

CHAPTER RESOURCES

1. Kochan, Jeffrey. "Vertebroplasty and Kyphoplasty, Percutaneous," eMedicine. http://emedicine.medscape.com/article/423209-overview. Accessed January 17, 2010.

2. Ibid.

3. Deramond, H., et al. 1998. Percutaneous vertebroplasty with polymethylmethacrylate. *Radiol Clin North Am* 36 (3): 533-46.

4. Kochan, Jeffrey. "Vertebroplasty and Kyphoplasty, Percutaneous," eMedicine. http://emedicine.medscape.com/article/423209-overview. Accessed January 17, 2010.

5. Buchbinder, R. 2009. A randomized trial of vertebroplasty for painful osteoporotic vertebral fractures. *New England Journal of Medicine* 361:557-568.

6. Goodman, B. New studies raise doubts about the benefits of vertebroplasty. *Arthitis Today*, 2009.

7. Kallmes, D.F., et al. 2009. A randomized trial of vertebroplasty for osteoporotic spinal fractures. *New England Journal of Medicine* 361 (6): 569-79.

8. Kulkarni, Shantanu. Spinal Orthotics. eMedicine. http://emedicine.medscape.com/article/314921-overview. Accessed January 20, 2010.

9. Reiter, GT. Vertebral Fracture. eMedicine. http://eMedicine.medscape.com/article/248236-overview Accessed January 12, 2010.

10. Ibid.

11. American Academy of Orthopaedic Surgeons (AAOS). "Osteoporosis Tests," AAOS website. http://orthoinfo.aaos.org/topic.cfm?topic=A00413. Accessed January 17, 2010.

12. NIH. "Osteoporosis," www.nlm.nih.gov/medlineplus/osteoporosis.html. Accessed January 17, 2010.

13. Mayo Clinic staff. "Exercising with osteoporosis: Stay active the safe way," MayoClinic.com. www.mayoclinic.com/print/osteoporosis/HQ00643/. Accessed January 17, 2010.

14. "Spinal Compression Fractures." www.eorthopod.com/node/10860. Accessed January 20, 2010.

Q & A *with Dr. Murinson*

Can I exercise after spinal fracture?

Exercise after spinal fracture, once you've been cleared for this by your doctor, is critically important for staying healthy and avoiding additional problems.[11] You should choose the exercise that you do based upon what is safe for your back, but also chose to do something that you enjoy. For some, exercise is an opportunity to engage in social interactions: Social exercisers can enjoy dancing, taking fitness classes, walking with a friend, or working out at the gym. Sometimes, exercise provides a time to be more focused on oneself. People who are pulled in many directions can find a few moments of contemplation in activities such as swimming, lifting weights at home, working out with headphones, or going to the gym very early in the morning.

It's important to choose your exercise with safety in mind. If you have osteoporosis or another condition that places you at risk for additional vertebral fractures, you may need to avoid exercises that require higher impacts or bending and twisting movements.[12] Examples of these include tennis, golf, rowing machines, and running.[13] Exercise bicycles are not considered ideal for the prevention of osteoporosis, as the exercise they provide is not weight-bearing. However, they are exceptionally good at promoting cardiovascular fitness while increasing strength and flexibility of the legs. For this reason, an exercise bike can be an excellent complement to other exercise activities that specifically target bone building.

What if I still have pain in my back after five weeks?

If your pain is gradually decreasing from the time of your injury but is lingering on at five weeks, you probably need to hang in there and anticipate that slow, steady improvement will be the name of the game.

If, however, your back pain is getting worse or changing for the worse quite suddenly, you may need to let your doctor know this is happening. If you're still getting physical therapy at five weeks after injury, ask your therapist what his or her sense of your recovery is. Vertebral fractures repair slowly, but the goal is to finish up with a stable spine that will allow you to return to everyday life and the activities you enjoy.[14]

CHAPTER 9

Syndromes of Spinal Cord Compression: Emergency!

Cancer or severe infection are rare but do occur.

Don't delay proper diagnosis and treatment.

the DIAGNOSIS

> Have you recently developed back pain, or has your mild back pain suddenly gotten much worse?

> Have your legs become weak, or are you recently having trouble getting to the bathroom without soiling or accidents?

If you have back pain with leg weakness or bowel or bladder incontinence, you need to seek immediate medical attention. Leg weakness and/or incontinence are considered red flags in the context of new or worsened back pain, as these symptoms can signal problems with the spinal cord or spinal roots. These kinds of problems when presenting together are not infrequently due to serious problems like cancer, aggressive infections, or problems with blood flow to the spine. To be sure, plenty of people have urinary incontinence for other reasons, such as prostate enlargement or pelvic floor problems after childbirth. But for someone who previously did not have these concerns to suddenly find themselves without good control over bodily functions, this is a cause for prompt assessment.

The treatments prescribed will depend on the identified cause of the problem. Although the causes of spinal cord compression are typically quite serious, if the problem is caught within a few hours of it starting, good treatment options may be available. Everything here depends on timing, though. Get help immediately.

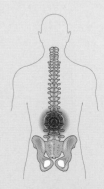

the PRESCRIPTION

If you have spinal cord compression in the neck:
- Your doctor will have determined the particular cause of spinal cord compression on the basis of X-rays and potentially other imaging studies (CT, MRI).
- Your neck may need to be immobilized or surgically fused.

If you have spinal cord compression in the middle of the back (thoracic region):
- Your doctor will have determined the particular cause of your spinal cord compression using a variety of tests. Blood tests, fluid samples, X-rays, MRIs, and CT scans may all be used.
- You may need to take medication for pain.
- Your doctor will discuss with you any procedures that will be required to stabilize the spine.

If you have spinal cord or root compression in the lower back (lumbar region and sacrum): Your doctor will have determined the particular cause of your compression syndrome on the basis of X-rays and other testing.
- Your doctor may recommend surgery to stabilize the spine. Depending on the specifics of the situation, spinal fusion may be required.
- You may need to take medication for pain.
- You may be instructed to eliminate certain activities for several weeks if spine surgery is needed.

The Treatment

Depending on the causes of spinal cord compression, treatments may vary from emergency surgery to medications to radiation. Make sure that you ask questions along the way and let your providers know immediately if new problems develop.

IDENTIFY A SUPPORT PERSON BEFORE SURGERY

If your doctor says you have to undergo surgery, make sure that you understand the nature and expected outcome of the planned procedure. Things may move very quickly if you have cord compression, so you'll want to have your family members or close ones aware of what is happening. You will be unconscious for the surgery, and your surgeon may have important information to communicate to you after the surgery. You will want to have someone present as much of the time as possible, just to help get through the first few hours and days of this process. It would be a good idea to have a designated family spokesperson. This should be someone who understands your personal opinions about healthcare and can speak for you. Ideally, this person should be comfortable talking to doctors, nurses, and social workers. The legal structure that exists to support this is the healthcare power of attorney. The laws pertaining to this vary by state, but be aware that the best decisions usually follow a willingness to be proactive about making sure your medical wishes are known and represented.

DIFFERENT TYPES OF SURGERY

The use of surgery for spinal cord compression will vary depending on the nature of the problem. If the problem is a tumor of the spinal cord itself and the tumor is still relatively small, surgery itself may be curative.[2] The limitation here is that tumors of the spinal cord itself are often discovered fairly late, after the tumor has grown in size and is damaging delicate structures. In the case of a focal infection such as an epidural abscess, the treatment may require a combination of medications and surgery.[3] In this situation, surgery is used to drain any pus and to stabilize the spine if needed.

ASK ABOUT SIDE EFFECTS OF MEDICATIONS

If your doctor says you need powerful medications, the type of medication will depend on the nature of the problem. For some problems, steroids may be used; for other situations, strong antibiotics may be necessary. Make sure to ask about expected side effects and whether there are any symptoms that might be especially worrisome and that doctors would want to know about right away.

What's New: Steroids within Eight Hours of Compression

For many years, the urgent treatment of spinal cord compression included the administration of high-dose steroid medications. The medications, although helpful in certain circumstances, are associated with serious side effects like bleeding from the stomach or intestines, transient diabetes, weight gain, thinning of the bones, atrophy of muscles, and increased skin fragility. Large-scale studies have indicated that steroids are only demonstrably beneficial when given very early after the onset of an injury to the spinal cord. Current recommendations indicate that eight hours is the time window during which steroids may be helpful, but leave it to the discretion of the treating doctor to proceed or not.[1]

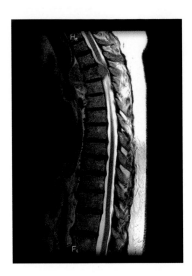

▲ MRI image of a metastatic tumor mass in the upper thoracic spinal canal and causing compression of the underlying spinal cord.

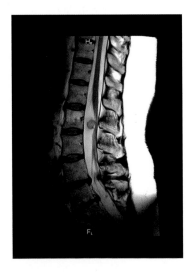

▲ MRI image of a neurofibroma.

EXPECTATIONS FOR REHABILITATION

If your doctor recommends rehabilitation, ask about what his or her expectations are for rehabilitation. Do people with your condition expect to make a full recovery, or are the problems persistent? Rehab for spinal cord compression can go quickly if the compression was minor and brief, but when the compression is more serious and persists for more than a few hours, rehab can require months of hard work. Hours of exercises, learning to walk safely, and keeping one's balance will be part of the rehab plan.

Testing For Spinal Cord Compression

Testing for spinal cord compression will most typically occur in an emergency room setting, at least initially. Your doctor will want to make a detailed examination of the nervous system's functioning, especially with regard to functioning of the legs and the bowels. A digital rectal exam may be performed as part of this. Images of the back will be obtained; this may include X-rays, CT scans, and MRIs. Each of these imaging techniques has particular strengths, and all three may be used at some point. CT scans can be very valuable in terms of visualizing the bones of the back in detail. MRI is usually needed to assess structures such as masses, nerves, muscles, joint capsules, and ligaments. Under certain circumstances, other imaging methods will later be used to help assess whatever process led to the cord compression to start with.

The Explanation

Syndromes of spinal cord compression are divided into three main classes as follows:

1. extradural, meaning those that press on the spinal cord from outside the spinal canal
2. intradural-extramedullary, meaning those that compress the spinal cord from outside of the cord itself but from inside the spinal sac
3. intramedullary, meaning they arise from inside the structure of the spinal cord.[4]

The course of back pain in these different classes will vary. In the case of compressions that are due to problems within the spinal cord, the pain that results may start very gradually and remain vaguely defined in terms of location until the problem is quite advanced. A loss of sexual function may be the first sign of a real problem. Compressive problems that start outside the spinal cord may first press on a nerve root; in this case, the pain will be very specific to the level of the spine that is involved. If not addressed immediately however, the localizing nerve pain may ease off as the nerve is completely disabled and pain may progress to a deeper, bony type pain as the vertebral bones are involved.

The causes of spinal cord compression are multiple. Cancer is an important cause; spinal cord compression can be due to local tumors or to tumors that have spread from elsewhere in the body.[5] Certain tumors have a tendency to spread to the spinal column (the vertebral bones) and from there extend to the point of compressing the spine. These spine compression syndromes may be characterized by a period of nagging back pain that suddenly evolves to include leg weakness or incontinence. The cancers that follow this pattern most often are those of lung, breast, and prostate. To restore or preserve function and minimize pain, it is important to get help immediately. There are several treatments that can be used to reduce the effects of these tumors and to control any resulting pain.

Another type of cancer that causes spinal cord compression are tumors that arise directly from the spinal cord itself (cord tumors). These tumors include the ependymomas, the astrocytomas, and the hemangioblastomas.[6] Of these, the ependymomas are more common in adults, but even these are uncommon, with an estimated occurrence of less than one in 100,000 persons. The usual location for the cord tumors is in the neck, where they can affect functions of the lower body as well as causing weakness in the arms. The pain caused by cord tumors may come on very gradually. Problems caused by cord tumors develop so slowly that a patient typically has had some symptoms for two years at the time of diagnosis. The hallmark of pain from these tumors is that the pain is worse at night as the person is lying on their back. Most patients have some weakness prior to diagnosis, but sexual dysfunction and urinary incontinence may be the problems that prompt a patient to seek medical attention. In the case of ependymomas, the tumor may be growing within a capsule or covering. Removal of these sorts of tumors is curative. There are circumstances where spinal tumors are more aggressive, however, so it is important to wait for the pathologist's report before reaching any conclusions.

In some cases, spinal cord compression is caused by an infection. The infection can come from another part of the body: urinary tract infections, lung infections, skin abscesses, and implanted devices are potential sources of infection. Recent surgery, dental procedures, interventional procedures that require catheters or needles, and spinal injections are possible contributory factors as well. People with underlying immunodeficiency are at increased risk, as are alcoholics and those using IV drugs. People with diabetes have increased risk for all kinds of

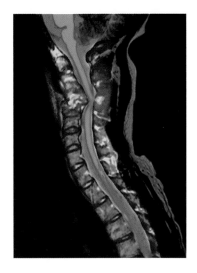

▲ MRI image of collapsing and inflammed spinal structures.

137

infections including epidural abscesses. The traditional picture of spinal abscess is that of a patient with fever, back pain, and neurological problems, but this is not always evident in each patient. The average age of patients with spinal abscess is surprisingly high, being around age 50.[7] Because of the seriousness of this infection, other systems of the body can become destabilized and a state of shock can follow.

This condition is a medical emergency. Both surgery and medical treatments may be used depending on the circumstances. Medications for a typical abscess due to bacterial infection may continue for four weeks or more. In years past, tuberculosis was a cause of spinal cord compression, but this is very rare in the U.S. at this time. The treatment for tumors that are pressing on the spinal cord from outside the spinal covering (dura) will depend on the tumor type and the extent of damage. In some cases, where vertebral bones are partially destroyed, a spinal fusion is needed. This procedure was described in detail in Chapter 7.

CHAPTER RESOURCES

1. Schreiber, Donald. "Spinal Cord Injuries: Treatment and Medication," eMedicine. http://emedicine. medscape.com/article/793582-treatment. Accessed March 16, 2010.

2. Ogden, Alfred, Nicholas Wetjen, and Thomas Francavilla. "Intramedullary Spinal Cord Tumors," eMedicine. http://emedicine.medscape.com/article/251133-overview. Accessed January 31, 2010.

3. Huff, Stephen. "Spinal Epidural Abscess," eMedicine. http://emedicine.medscape.com/ article/1165840-overview. Accessed January 31, 2010.

4. Dickman, Curtis, Michael Fehlings, and Ziya Gokaslan. *Spinal Cord and Spinal Column Tumors: Principles and Practice*. New York: Thieme, 2006.

5. Schick, U., G. Marquardt, and R. Lorenz. Intradural and extradural spinal metastases. *Journal Neurosurgical Review*, 2001, 24(1):1–5.

6. Ogden, Alfred, Nicholas Wetjen, and Thomas Francavilla. "Intramedullary Spinal Cord Tumors," eMedicine. http://emedicine.medscape.com/article/251133-overview. Accessed January 31, 2010.

7. Huff, Stephen. "Spinal Epidural Abscess," eMedicine. http://emedicine.medscape.com/ article/1165840-overview. Accessed January 31, 2010.

Q & A *with Dr. Murinson*

When will there be a cure for spinal cord injury?

Scientists are working furiously to find treatments that reverse the effects of spinal cord injury. Until recently, there was little hope of recovery for people with damaged spinal cords, but the future holds much promise. Scientific research has uncovered biological responses that actually interfere with the ability of the spinal cord to recover from an injury, and scientists are devising new strategies to promote effective healing and regrowth. The fundamental challenge is that the spinal cord serves as a conduit for nerve processes (axons) that extend from the base of the spine to the brain, sometimes over three feet (91 cm) in length. When these connections are damaged or even severed, it is not simply a matter of restoring the connection at the injury site; the axons actually have to grow from that point onwards to where they used to terminate, find the appropriate target and re-establish functional communications. To accomplish this would be a task of profound complexity. From studies of lab animals, we know that if the goal is being able to walk a bit, it's not actually necessary to restore all the original circuits. In rats at least, a few pioneer axons are enough to bring back some walking function. Although repair of human spinal cord injury remains a tantalizing goal, and some intractable mysteries are beginning to unravel, effective treatments remain just over the horizon. If you know someone with a spinal cord injury, and you want to get the latest on cutting-edge (experimental) treatments, visit the clinicaltrials.gov website and enter the search term "spinal cord injury."

Are there any other conditions that present like a spinal cord compression?

Occasionally, what appears to be a spinal cord compression syndrome is actually a spinal cord stroke. The blood supply to the spine is mainly carried by two large arteries: one that forms at the top of the spine in the neck and another that penetrates the spinal column in the mid-to-lower back. Blockage of either of these arteries or their major branches will have severe consequences including some pain, paralysis, incontinence, and sometimes loss of sensation. In this case, an immediate intervention to restore blood flow may be the only chance to provide meaningful recovery.

CHAPTER 10

Scoliosis

Early diagnosis and regular re-evaluation

is the key to a good outcome.

the DIAGNOSIS

> Are you (or do you know) a young person with a curvature of the spine from side to side?

> Does your back ache on most days of the week?

Scoliosis is a side-to-side curvature of the spine that usually affects young people in the mid-teen to early adult years. Girls are more often affected than boys. The common scenarios for scoliosis include chronic daily back pain, feelings of fatigue, and some shortness of breath. Scoliosis shows up as a difference in shoulder height, an obvious curvature of the spine, or something more subtle, such as a need to adjust a bra strap to be shorter on one side.[1] Early treatment of scoliosis is important for good outcomes.

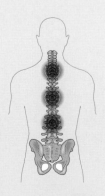

the PRESCRIPTION

Back pain due to scoliosis needs expert medical assessment and care. Because this problem occurs most commonly in adolescence, most pediatricians are familiar with the screening procedures. If scoliosis is suspected on the basis of the physical exam, usually an X-ray will be needed. There are special methods for measuring the degree of curvature of the spine. The treatment depends on how severely the spine is curving and whether the curvature is getting worse quickly. Most commonly, scoliosis develops between the ages of 10 and 14. Exact numbers aren't known, but most studies find that girls are 10 times more often affected than boys. If surgery is needed, there is a preference for delaying the surgery if possible until after the last growth spurt so that there will be no need for later revision.

If you have mild scoliosis:
- Your doctor will very likely recommend physical therapy, especially if there is no evidence that the curvature of the spine is rapidly worsening. The effectiveness of physical therapy for scoliosis depends both on the type of exercises prescribed and on the consistency of the person following the exercise recommendations.
- Your doctor will want to re-evaluate your spine in the next few months.

If you have moderate scoliosis:
- Your doctor will very likely recommend fitting for a brace. Bracing is widely used to stabilize the spine and prevent worsening of scoliosis in situations where there is moderate curvature of the spine. In order to be effective, the brace must be worn nearly all the time. It is important to have the brace reassessed for fit at intervals as the person wearing the brace will be growing and adjustment may be necessary.
- Again, your doctor will want to re-evaluate your spine in the next few months.

If you have more severe scoliosis:

- Your doctor may recommend assessment for surgery. Depending on the overall medical picture, surgery is currently recommended for scoliosis where there is a more substantial curvature to the spine. The risks of leaving severe scoliosis untreated include chronic pain, breathing problems, and risks for infection.
- Your doctor may recommend a brace for a period of time to allow for a growth period to be completed prior to surgical intervention. Although surgery may eventually still be needed, the results of surgery are often more favorable if growth is completed or nearly so.
- Make sure that you discuss the risks and benefits of surgery thoroughly before proceeding. What are the expectations for relief of pain? How straight will the spine be after surgery? Will future surgery be needed?

What if your doctor diagnoses a specific problem causing the scoliosis?
In this case, the treatment may depend on whether that specific cause of scoliosis is reversible or curable. In rare cases, there may be a tumor, infection, or other abnormality that is inducing the curvature in the spine (secondary scoliosis).

Geography Is a Factor

The percentage of young people developing scoliosis varies with geographic location. There is a tendency for people from more northern countries to develop more scoliosis. It is believed that there is an effect from sun exposure (or lack of it) and possible effects in those with later puberty to be more at risk. Whatever the mechanism, the occurrence of scoliosis in the U.S. is reported to range from 2 to 5 percent in girls aged 10 to 14.[2]

High Risk for Surgical Complications

Ask your surgeon to provide specific details about the rate of complication in their surgery practice. It is recognized that surgery for scoliosis carries a relatively high complication rate.[6] In addition to the usual concerns associated with a major spine surgery, such as blood loss and infection, surgery for scoliosis carries certain neurological risks and over the long run may increase the rate of degenerative spine disease at levels above and below the area of stabilized spine. It is known that more aggressive efforts to fully reduce spine curvature are associated with added stress on nearby structures. For this reason, spinal surgery for scoliosis does not seek to attain a perfect result. The long-term consequences could be quite negative. Some of the risks associated with scoliosis surgery are more pronounced in young people who have scoliosis as a result of an underlying nerve or muscle disease (neuromuscular disease), such as myopathy or muscular dystrophy. Most of the patients with idiopathic scoliosis are otherwise healthy and would be considered good candidates for surgery.

The Treatment

If your doctor recommends physical therapy first, this usually means that you have a mild or early form of scoliosis. It is very important to pursue physical therapy with a commitment to making this work, as a failure of physical therapy usually means moving on to more expensive, uncomfortable, and cumbersome treatments such as a brace that is worn full-time or a major spine surgery.

PHYSICAL THERAPY REDUCES THE CURVATURE

The essential goal of physical therapy is to reduce the curvature of the spine. This is usually done with exercises that strengthen the spine. One approach, called Scientific Exercises Approach to Scoliosis (SEAS), teaches patients to recognize the location of their most pronounced spine curvature and actively learn how to reduce this curvature intentionally.[3] This requires a training period wherein the patient is assisted by a treatment specialist who assists in this process of neuromuscular training. The patient then performs a series of exercises while consciously correcting the areas of curvature. This is referred to as *active self-correction*. Other approaches to physical therapy involve stretching frames and exercise equipment to reduce the curvature of the spine more passively in response to certain postures or exercises.[4] The benefits of physical therapy are debated by some but there is accumulating evidence that certain forms may be demonstrable benefits.[5]

A BRACE FOR MODERATE SCOLIOSIS

If your doctor recommends a brace, this usually means you have a moderate or gradually progressive form of scoliosis. There is widespread agreement that for bracing to be effective, the brace must be worn all day with short breaks for bathing and other selected activities. The brace needs to be worn to bed at night and should be comfortable enough that it can be worn during the school day and to all social activities. Some specialists recommend 23 hours of brace wearing daily, but check with your provider to determine their specific instructions.

Scoliosis braces come in different forms. The most traditional is a hard plastic brace that fits around the waist and extends upward to the underarms and down to the hips as required for the specific spine curvature. The rigid brace is usually made out of white plastic and is strapped to the body. Because it extends down to the hips, it is important to have it checked for fit so hip growth is not impeded. The brace can be fit from a modular system such as the Boston brace or custom manufactured by a local prosthestist. Another brace type consists of elastic straps and a pelvic stabilization belt; it may require bands that wrap around the upper thigh and groin.

SURGERY FOR SEVERE SCOLIOSIS

If your doctor recommends surgery, this usually means you have a more severe or frankly progressive form of scoliosis. The surgery for scoliosis usually involves the placement of rods in certain sections of the spine to partially correct the curvature of the spine. When scoliosis is severe, there is danger of neurological effects such as compression of the spinal cord or nerves. Breathing problems may develop, leading to recurrent pneumonia, and repeated infections can have life-threatening consequences. Lifelong poor body mechanics and serious chronic pain can develop.

In light of these negatives, the effects of surgery may seem minimal but it is important not to underestimate the impact of major spinal surgery. A fair number of patients have some persistent pain after surgery. Usually this pain is described as mild-to-moderate, rating about 3 out of 10 points, on average. The cumulative effects of daily mild pain are not known but are not positive in any case. The spine will never bend normally once spinal rods are in place. This is a consequence that must be accepted. It is probably prudent to exercise some care in the choice of physical activities after the placement of spinal rods. Excessive stress on the rods may lead to loosening of the attachments with pain as a result.

Make sure that you discuss the specific plans for surgery with your surgeon beforehand. Know what to expect in terms of recovery time, time off from school, and impact of future activities. Ask if the rods will ever be removed and under what circumstances this might happen.

The procedures of surgery for scoliosis are essentially those of spinal fusion surgery, but may or may not include a bone-graft type fusion per se. One commonly performed surgery is referred to as *spinal fusion with instrumentation*. *Instrumentation* is the technical term for the hardware that is used to stabilize the spine. The general aspects of spinal fusion surgery are described in Chapter 7.

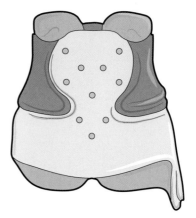

▲ Scoliosis braces are often custom-built for therapeutic effect and for comfort. The custom brace shown is made of multiple materials shown in white, light gray, and medium gray.

Testing For Scoliosis

Testing for scoliosis will initially take place in the primary care provider's office. The doctor, nurse, or PA will want to make an examination of the back and will need to see the how the back responds to movement, especially bending forward. Images of the back will be obtained; this typically includes special X-rays that visualize most of the spine from top to bottom. The radiologists will make a measurement of the curves in the spine and the numbers will be reported back to the referring provider.

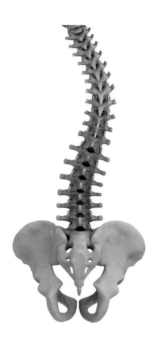

▲ Spine with scoliosis

The Explanation

Scoliosis is usually a condition of the spine that becomes problematic during the pre-teen and early teen years. The precise cause of most patients' scoliosis is unknown. It is more common in populations where puberty occurs later. One of the debated topics in the medical literature is the usefulness of large screening programs for scoliosis. The bottom line is that if a side-to-side curvature of the spine is significant enough that you have noticed it, it deserves evaluation.

Each form of scoliosis is unique, although common patterns are seen. A single curve scoliosis will be described as having a "C" shape; when a second curve appears, it is usually compensatory in nature and will cause an S-shaped curvature of the spine. A scoliosis will be named for the part of the spine that are most affected, described as being a right or left scoliosis based on whether the most pronounced part of the curve is to the right or left. Imagine an arrow pointing into the major curve and that arrow will point to the side that is used to label the scoliosis.

Although the most common form of scoliosis is idiopathic (meaning we don't know the cause), there are actually some forms of scoliosis that have specific causes. These might include a compensatory scoliosis due to a leg-length discrepancy, where the body tries to compensate for an angled pelvis with curvature of the spine. Rarely, tumors can induce a shape change in the spine; muscle spasm can cause the spine to curve to one side; and problems with the pelvis itself can cause a curvature.[7]

CHAPTER RESOURCES

1. Dreeden, Olga. *Introduction to Physical Therapy for Physical Therapist Assistants*. Sudbury, MA: Jones and Bartlett Publishers, 2007.

2. Grivas, T.B., et al. 2006. Association between adolescent idiopathic scoliosis prevalence and age at menarche in different geographic latitudes. *Scoliosis* 1:9.

3. Romano, M., et al. Scientific Exercises Approach to Scoliosis (SEAS): In *The Conservative Scoliosis Treatment*, T.B. Grivas, ed. Amsterdam: IOS Press, 2008.

4. Weiss, H.R. and A. Maier-Hennes. Specific exercises in the treatment of scoliosis. In *The Conservative Scoliosis Treatment*, T.B. Grivas, ed. Amsterdam: IOS Press, 2008.

5. Negrini, S., et al. 2008. Specific exercises reduce brace prescription in adolescent idiopathic scoliosis. *J Rehabil Med* 40 (6): 451-5.

6. Weiss, H.R., and D. Goodall. 2008. Rate of complications in scoliosis surgery: A systematic review of the Pub Med literature. *Scoliosis* 3:9.

7. Tecklin, Jan Stephen. *Pediatric Physical Therapy, Fourth Edition*. Philadelphia, PA: Lippincott Williams & Wilkins, 2007.

Is surgery the only way to treat scoliosis?

The treatment of scoliosis depends on the severity and progression of the abnormal curvatures of the spine. Scoliosis will sometimes respond to the use of a brace, but the brace must be worn for most of the day and night. This is awkward for some patients, particularly as scoliosis usually strikes at a time of life when issues surrounding body image are very important.

What happens if I don't treat the scoliosis?

In its mildest forms, scoliosis can be a self-resolving process, becoming milder as the person grows. In many cases however, untreated scoliosis worsens. It can lead to spinal collapse, chronic severe pain, breathing problems, and compression of vital organs. I once saw an active lady in her mid-thirties who had gradually worsening back pain and spasms. She'd been told that her nerves were the cause of the problem and was given heavy doses of muscle relaxants to take for this. Despite the use of multiple medications, her pain got to the point where she was limited to working three days a week. She was miserable in her marriage and felt that she was failing as a mother. She began to travel from doctor to doctor looking for a solution. She came to my clinic desperate for solutions and we began with a fresh evaluation. Although she'd been told as a young person that she had scoliosis, it seemed that none of the doctors who saw her as an adult had taken this seriously. At the time of her first visit with me, she was in nearly continuous muscle spasms and pain.

Her spine was curved from side to side with her shoulders and hips tilted at biomechanically unfavorable angles. We obtained new X-rays and a new MRI. The images showed a pronounced scoliosis of the thoracic and lumbar spine. In her lower back, one vertebra appeared to be slowly slipping off to the side and forward, compressing nerves and straining ligaments. This in itself probably accounted for her daily severe pain. Armed with the new information about her worsening scoliosis, she sought treatment from a local surgeon and ultimately did well. Although it was a joy to finally get this brave lady connected with a correct diagnosis and back on the path to a normal life, it was a pity that this could not have been properly treated earlier in life before her family and work activities were so severely disrupted.

CHAPTER 11

Spinal Stenosis

Medication, physical therapy, and exercise may help, but sometimes surgery is the best solution.

the DIAGNOSIS

> **Are you more than 60 years of age?**

> **Have you been finding that you can only walk or stand for so long before your back and legs begin to hurt?**

Many people find as they mature that the back is less resilient than it was in prior years. In part, this is because the discs of the back dry out starting in the mid-twenties and are remarkably less springy as time goes on. Other people find that they have one or two problem areas in their backs, perhaps an SI joint that tends to go out or a particular muscle strain that recurs from time to time. Still other people, especially those with an adventuresome spirit, will find that their back is just disabling them. They can barely walk, they wake up each morning with substantial pain, they sleep poorly at night, and they can't do most of the things they had looked forward to in retirement. If this sounds like you, then a diagnosis of spinal stenosis may be the explanation for your troubles.

Most people with spinal stenosis find that flexing the spine will relieve some of the symptoms. So if sitting down for a bit seems to make things better, this might be a sign that spinal stenosis is producing your symptoms. The classical sign of spinal stenosis, recognized by the old-time doctors, was that it was easier for people with this condition to walk uphill than down. This is because the spine flexes a bit as we walk uphill and extends as the pelvis tilts back to accommodate downhill walking.

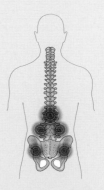

the *PRESCRIPTION*

What's New: Profile of Stenosis Patient

The last several years have seen a flurry of large clinical trials looking at spinal stenosis. Through these studies, a clearer picture of what spinal stenosis is and how to best treat it has emerged. The picture of the patient with stenosis is someone in their mid-sixties, tipping the scales at the high end of the overweight range, and possibly suffering with hypertension and some other arthritis. Women are slightly more likely to be affected.

The impact of spinal stenosis on quality of life is substantial, with bodily pain and inability to function causing more interference than limitations in mental function. People with spinal stenosis may still be working but more often are retired. The symptoms that predominate include difficulty with walking distances (pseudoclaudication) and pain that wraps around the leg from the buttock into the foot.[1]

Back pain due to spinal stenosis needs expert medical assessment and care. In mild cases, physical therapy may be used to relieve pain. Depending on the level of concern and local practice patterns, your doctor may want you to have some kind of injection. Surgery is beneficial for patients with moderate to severe stenosis.

If you have spinal stenosis:

- Your doctor may recommend physical therapy, especially if your disease is mild or there are reasons that surgery would not be feasible. The effectiveness of physical therapy for spinal stenosis depends on the skillfulness of the therapist, the degree of stenosis, and the motivation of the patient.
- Your doctor may recommend injection of the back with pain-active medications such as lidocaine or cortisone. These medications may provide temporary relief from pain and may allow the physical therapist a window of opportunity for more aggressive treatments, but injections such as these may not provide a lasting benefit.
- Your doctor may recommend that you have a surgical consultation for spinal decompression and fusion. This will depend on the severity of your spinal stenosis at this point and your overall medical picture.

WHAT IF YOUR DOCTOR DIAGNOSES A SLIPPED DISC?

In this case, you may still need surgery. Please see Chapter 2 on disc herniation.

WHAT IF YOUR DOCTOR FINDS THAT YOU HAVE SYMPTOMS OF SPINAL STENOSIS BUT NO EVIDENCE FOR IT ON MRI OR X-RAY?

The clinical description of spinal stenosis is someone who has difficulty with walking distances. It is sometimes possible to have problems like this from other causes. Possibilities include problems with the heart, problems with circulation of blood to the legs, and problems in other parts of the nervous system. If you are experiencing shortness of breath, you need to seek immediate medical attention. Especially if your pain is limited to the back of the calf and always comes on after walking a specific number of blocks, you should encourage your doctor to check out your leg circulation.

In rare cases, spinal stenosis is due to a mass (tumor), an infection (abscess), or a fracture. These serious but rare causes of spinal stenosis are usually assessed through the diagnostic tests described later in this chapter. The treatment for these conditions is individualized.

The Treatment

If your doctor recommends physical therapy first, this usually means that your spinal stenosis is not ideally treated with surgery at this time. If you have severe symptoms from spinal stenosis and surgery is not being considered, make sure you understand why. Does the doctor have particular health concerns that make surgery a poor option? Is there some aspect of your stenosis that precludes surgery, or does the doctor view your problem as not severe enough for a surgical referral?

PHYSICAL THERAPY IS WIDELY USED

Physical therapy is widely used as a treatment for spinal stenosis.[2] Several forms of physical therapy are effective for limiting the impact of spinal stenosis. In addition, I often encourage patients to pursue some physical therapy before surgery, depending on their circumstances. This is because surgery can be very demanding on the body and people who are in better physical condition can get through the process more easily. The types of physical therapy used for spinal stenosis can include thermal therapies, electrical stimulation, manual therapies, and conditioning and strengthening work.

Warning! Some Exercises Are Harmful

Avoid exercises that extend the spine; examples of this could include certain types of standing aerobic exercise machines. Arching the back (extending the spine) is likely to worsen the symptoms of spinal stenosis.

MANUAL THERAPIES EASE SYMPTOMS

Manual therapies such as massage and gentle spinal manipulation can provide some relief from the symptoms of spinal stenosis, especially if back pain is part of the overall symptoms. Sometimes, people with spinal stenosis don't have appreciable back pain, and sometimes people don't realize how much discomfort they did have until they get some treatment and start to feel better. Given that spinal stenosis is believed to result from an accumulation of minor injuries to the back over time, perhaps some people who develop spinal stenosis don't have very sensitive backs, and maybe they develop spinal stenosis because a lot of damage has occurred without much pain being experienced to slow them down and make them stop a harmful activity.

THERMAL THERAPIES ACCOMPANY PT

Particularly with spinal stenosis, it is important to prevent any strain or swelling of the low back structures. Warm compresses can help reduce muscle strain and promote relaxation. Ice packs will help to prevent and reduce swelling and can block pain signaling from the nearby structures. If you think a warm compress or an ice pack would help, make sure to ask your physical therapist if they haven't already offered it.

ELECTRICAL STIMULATION MIGHT IMPROVE BLOOD FLOW

Electrical stimulation may or may not be used, depending on the experience of your therapist and local practices. Electrical stimulation may be helpful for relaxing muscles and secondarily improving blood flow. It may or may not be beneficial with spinal stenosis.

STRENGTHENING AND CONDITIONING REQUIRES PROFESSIONAL GUIDANCE

The process of spinal stenosis can make sustained exercise more hazardous. Some recommended exercises include the use of an exercise bike, as the typical posture for this flexes the spine and should be better tolerated by someone with spinal stenosis.[3] Your physical therapist will have many good ideas for how you can improve your muscle strength and maintain your level of fitness even while living with spinal stenosis. You should do balance exercises, as they will help you avoid falls. Consciously trying to challenge and improve your balance will have positive effects.

One exercise that works well is the bent-knee sidestep. Check this out with your doctor or therapist first, but it works as follows. First find a place where you will have good support if you need to reach out and stabilize your stance. Often a hallway that is not too wide works well for this. Turn so that you are standing sideways in the hallway and place your feet about shoulder-width apart. Bend your knees slightly and tuck your tail bone; tighten your stomach muscles and hold them tightened throughout the exercise or as long as you can. To begin the exercise, lift your right foot and take a sidestep of about six to nine inches (15 to 23 cm) to the right. As your weight transfers to the right, bring your left foot over with a matching step. Take four more steps to the right, moving slowly until you are more confident with this process. Maintain your balance and try to distribute your weight evenly between your two feet in between steps. Now take five steps to the left. Repeat this exercise three more times back and forth.

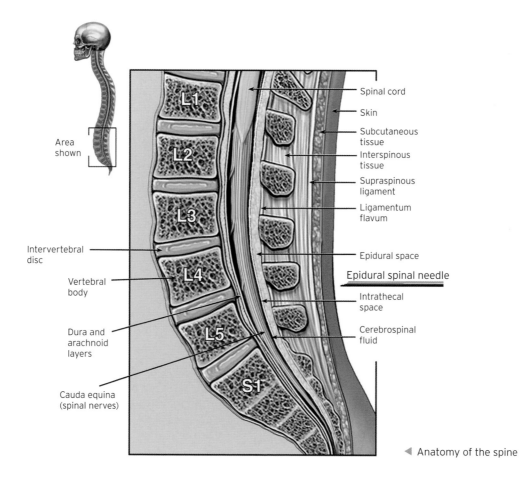

Area shown

Spinal cord

Skin

Subcutaneous tissue

Interspinous tissue

Supraspinous ligament

Ligamentum flavum

Intervertebral disc

Vertebral body

Epidural space

Epidural spinal needle

Intrathecal space

Dura and arachnoid layers

Cerebrospinal fluid

Cauda equina (spinal nerves)

◀ Anatomy of the spine

Another exercise that can help support balance and is accomplishable while maintaining a flexed spine position comes from the dance world. Stand in a place where you can reach out for support if necessary. Begin by standing on two feet, with your feet about 10 inches (25 cm) apart, wider if needed for stability. Bend your knees slightly as you tuck your tailbone. Transferring your weight to your right foot, lift your left foot and swing it gently to the side and bring it back as you maintain balance on the right foot. Continue to swing your left foot out to the side and back to center several more times. Then switch your stance to the left foot and move the right leg out and back. This exercise provides a good dynamic challenge to the ankle muscles. It will strengthen them without overly taxing your back and doesn't require any special equipment.

PAIN INJECTIONS PROVIDE IMMEDIATE RELIEF

If your doctor recommends treatment with a pain injection, this may provide some immediate relief—but it may not be a lasting solution. Usually, pain injections are performed using a mixture of fast-acting local anesthetic and a steroid to reduce pain over the longer term. While these injections can provide immediate relief, they do carry certain risks, such as a small riskof infection and longer-range risks of problems associated with steroid use.These injections are a way to make someone who is in terrible pain comfortable more quickly, and occasionally someone will have a dramatic and lasting improvement in response to an injection or two. Most of the time, however, these injections can only be repeated a few times and they are not a good long-term solution to spinal stenosis.

ORAL MEDICINES DULL THE PAIN

Many medications can be used for the treatment of pain related to spinal stenosis. The specific choice of medication will depend on the type and suspected cause of the pain. If your pain is due to compression of specific nerve roots, your doctor may recommend prescription medication. If it seems that arthritis or inflammation is a major part of your pain, then an over-the-counter or prescription anti-inflammatory medication (NSAID) may be prescribed. Long-term drug therapy is likely in the treatment of spinal stenosis. If opioids are used, address the potential for constipation even before treatment starts. Make sure to keep these medications stored safely, especially if there are other people coming and going in your home.

Each medication will have specific side effects. If antidepressants are used, they can include weight gain, sleepiness, bizarre feelings, delay in urinary function, or a loss of libido. Some people will experience no side effects, while others will not be able to take even a small dose of medicine. At this point in time, the only predictor of whether a medication will cause troublesome side effects is your prior experience with it, so it is often helpful to keep a brief journal about your pain and its treatment. If NSAIDs are used, ask your doctor about something to protect your stomach. Some European doctors routinely prescribe an additional medicine to protect against gastric bleeding with NSAIDs. If you doctor isn't comfortable adding an extra medication, discuss it with your pharmacist, who may have some good recommendations.

While oral medications will probably help with the pain, it is quite possible that other steps will be necessary to address the limitations of spinal stenosis. Oral pain medicines will have limited effect on the compression of nerve roots and restrictions on local blood flow that result from spinal stenosis.

SURGERY IS RECOMMENDED FOR SEVERE STENOSIS

Surgery may well be the best treatment for spinal stenosis, depending on the disease severity and your other medical conditions. Recent clinical research has compared standard medical management of spinal stenosis with spine fusion surgery and found that surgery has better results in terms of pain, function, and patient satisfaction. Spinal fusion surgery is a serious undertaking (see Chapter 7 for details), but people with moderate-to-severe spinal stenosis can be so limited in terms of activity and quality of life that the surgery is worthwhile. The usual surgery for spinal stenosis is lumbar decompression and fusion. Decompression is the process of removing built-up portions of bone and sometimes removing the roof of the spinal canal. This is done to relieve pressure on transiting nerves and nerve roots and is part of the overall surgery.

Testing for Spinal Stenosis

The diagnosis of spinal stenosis can often be made clinically on the basis of your recent medical history and the examination in the office. However, since most advanced cases of spinal stenosis need to be evaluated for surgical intervention, it is important to know that imaging with both MRI and X-ray may be required. In some situations, it may be necessary to include other tests as well. This is because spinal stenosis is a complex disorder that shares aspects with other causes of back pain. Your doctor may also order a nerve conduction test to better define the extent of any possible nerve damage. (See Chapter 2.) Once all the test results are in, a clearer picture will emerge. The possibilities range from "nothing is clearly wrong" to "moderate spine degeneration" to "severe degeneration of the spine."

Warning!
Put a Lock on It

Opioids as a group, although generally safe when taken as your doctor prescribes, are subject to a growing problem of prescription drug use among young people aged 18 to 25. The 2008 U.S. national study showed that nearly 5 percent of young adults have tried pain reliever medications that were not prescribed to them, most illegally obtained from friends or family.[4]

What's New: Surgery Produces Good Results

The latest studies are now reporting on the multi-year follow-up from the initial favorable reports of surgery, and these longer term results continue to favor surgery when possible and appropriate.[5]

The Explanation

Spinal stenosis, in its most common form, is an advanced degeneration of the spine where progressive compression of the vertebral discs, accumulated traumas to the joints, overgrowth of the bones from repeated strains, and enlargement of the ligaments all come together to make smooth passage of the nerves to and from the spinal cord impossible. In spinal stenosis, the back is functioning at a permanent mechanical disadvantage. Ongoing arthritis and inflammation create a vicious cycle of persistent pain, and compressed nerves fire off pain signals that worsen with every step. For years, medical doctors have been trying to treat spinal stenosis they best they know how. Medicines, physical therapy, heating pads, aqua therapy, braces, sometimes even walkers are used to relieve pressure on the spine. A recent landmark study indicated that surgical interventions, if a person is in good health to tolerate a major spine surgery, may have the best chance of helping patients make a meaningful recovery. Some of the major specialists in the field indicate that people with spinal stenosis may or may not have much back pain.

CHAPTER RESOURCES

1. Weinstein, et al. 2007. Surgical versus nonsurgical treatment for lumbar degenerative spondylolisthesis. *N Engl J Med* 356 (22): 2257-70.

2. Weinstein, J.N., et al. 2007. Surgical versus nonsurgical treatment for lumbar degenerative spondylolisthesis. *N Engl J Med* 356 (22): 2257-70.

3. Reed, Stephen, Penny Kendall-Reed, Michael Ford, and Charles Gregory. *The Complete Doctor's Healthy Back Bible*. Toronto: Robert Rose, Inc., 2004.

4. "Results from the 2008 National Survey on Drug Use and Health: National Findings," U.S. Department of Health and Human Services, Substance Abuse and Mental Health Services Administration, Office of Applied Studies. http://www.oas.samhsa.gov/nsduh/2k8nsduh/2k8Results. cfm. Accessed February 9, 2010.

5. Weinstein, J.N., et al. 2009. Surgical compared with nonoperative treatment for lumbar degenerative spondylolisthesis: Four-year results in the Spine Patient Outcomes Research Trial (SPORT) randomized and observational cohorts. *J Bone Joint Surg Am* 91 (6): 1295-304.

What causes spinal stenosis?

The spine is an engineering miracle, and most of us experience years of good, productive service from our backs with minimal effort. Spinal stenosis is usually the result of many years of moderate strain on the back, sometimes punctuated by specific traumas: A fall from a horse, a car accident, that time you pulled the lawnmower up a flight of stairs, shoveling snow, moving furniture, a bike accident, and gardening all add up to a lifetime of insults to the back. Over time, the back responds in several ways. The discs compress down to a fraction of their original height, dramatically narrowing the space available for nerves to enter and exit the spine and, at the same time, reducing the biomechanics of spine movement. The discs will often bulge out, which might not be so bad, but the ligaments and facet joints on the back side of the spinal canal are enlarging at the same time. It's kind of mysterious, but part of our biological nature is not unlike bricks and stone that wear away with time and pressure, our bones and ligaments respond to stress and strain by overgrowing or hypertrophying. If you have spinal stenosis or advancing spinal degeneration, and you are able to get a hold of your MRI report, you may read terms such as "ligamentous hypertrophy," "facet joint enlargement," or "narrowing of the neural foramina." All of these are terms that the radiologist will use to describe the basic disease components that together make up spinal stenosis.

CHAPTER 12

Coccydynia

Manage coccydynia pain by reducing stressful activities, using a cushion, and losing excess body weight.

> **Do you have pain at the bottom end of your spine?**

> **Does your pain get substantially worse the longer you sit on a hard surface?**

People with coccydynia know a special misery. These are the patients who pace the waiting room, carrying their donut cushion and wincing every time someone asks them to take a seat. The pain of coccydynia is centered at the very bottom of the spine, deep in the crease of the buttocks. Although small and tucked away inside the body, the tailbone serves an essential function as an anchor for ligaments and muscles in the buttock and rectum area.

Although the cause of coccydynia is not always identified, it can certainly arise from a trauma such as a slip-fall type accident, such as landing hard on your bottom while ice skating. When a specific causative injury is identified, the chances of recovery may be even better than when the syndrome occurs without a definable cause, although the reason for this is unknown.

Coccydynia Aggravators

- Bicycling
- Sitting on a stadium bench
- Horseback riding
- Jarring carnival rides
- Motorcycle riding
- Unicycle riding (!)
- Childbirth

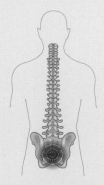

the PRESCRIPTION

Dealing with Pain while Sitting

Leaning forward while sitting transfers weight away from the tailbone and onto the sitz bones, while leaning back increases the pressures of sitting. For this reason, people with coccydynia will often naturally lean forward when they must sit. There are specialized chairs that have been used by people with coccydynia. While not especially portable, these chairs may normalize life at home and work.

Coccydynia pain is usually increased during the moment of transition from sitting to standing. This is when the mechanical stresses are focused on the tailbone. You may need to let people know that you'll need to stand during meetings.

The first major goal is to avoid re-injury of the tip of your spine. It is important to take all reasonable precautions not to fall; this may sound silly, but take extra care when walking. Avoid activities where falls and trauma are likely, including skating, skiing, motorcycle riding, tractors, school buses, and amusement park rides. Especially if you are healing from such an injury, special care is needed.

You will probably need to combine medication and non-medication treatments to get through an episode of coccydynia. Medications can include NSAIDs, acetaminophen, or prescription pain medications. Non-medication treatments will certainly include using a cushion but may also include stretches, manual therapy, hot and cold packs, and any of the non-medication therapies discussed in the second part of this book.

- Reducing inflammation will aid in control of coccydynia. Your tools for reducing inflammation will include rest (as appropriate), ice, and anti-inflammatory medications (NSAIDs). Your doctor may recommend the injection of an anti-inflammatory medicine such as a steroid. This can be helpful if everything goes well. Consider your options carefully.
- You will need to buy and carry a cushion. The donut is the most common but there are other types of cushions that relieve pressure on the coccyx. Coccydynia is usually worsened by pressure on the buttock while sitting. You need to think before agreeing to go someplace unfamiliar and determine if an extra cushion will carry you through. Some activities, like sporting events that take place in a stadium with bench seating, are best avoided until a recovery is made.
- People who are overweight or obese place added strain on the tailbone and for this reason, weight control may be recommended when appropriate.
- Constipation is another aggravator of coccydynia, so make sure to stay well hydrated and have an active treatment regimen (fiber, laxative) to prevent constipation.

The Treatment

Pain control for coccydynia will proceed along the lines of therapy for many other conditions: first, heat and cold therapies are used. Sometimes electrical stimulation is considered and some practitioners will apply ultrasound or try iontophoresis of medications through the skin. On occasion, manipulation of the tailbone will be tried; however, support for this in the medical literature is limited.[1] One older clinical report suggests that manual manipulation in combination with injection is more effective than either method alone.[2]

DONUT CUSHIONS REDUCE THE PRESSURE

If your doctor tells you that you need a cushion, you will probably be advised to start with a donut. Donut cushions are named for their shape; they look like giant donuts. The rationale of the donut is that it will reduce the pressure on the tailbone and thereby alleviate pain. They may work for some people, but not everyone will respond as well. Sometimes the cushion is not firm enough and doesn't take enough of the pressure off the tailbone. Other times the donut cushion just doesn't feel right; it might cause pressure points elsewhere in the buttock. The other parts of the body that bears most of the weight when we're seated are the sitz bones, more formally called the *ischial tuberosities*. Each of the bony spots in the buttock are cushioned with a fluid-filled sac called a bursa. There are many bursas in the body and they are usually found at points of mechanical stress. They are great when they work: the bursas in the shoulder allow smooth gliding movements even when someone is lifting a heavy load. The problem is that bursas can become inflamed, and when they do, look out—it's a whole new cause of pain that can compound an already difficult situation.

The donut can irritate the bursas in the buttock, so many people use other types of cushions: there are triangular wedge cushions that have a cut-out along the back edge to relieve tailbone pressure, and there are fancy commercial cushions with a groove down the middle, designed to relieve midline buttock and pelvic pressures. For most people, any cushion is better than none, and the worst situation is where someone is compelled to sit for long periods on a hard surface. This can occur a lot in the spring when students are graduating, or during sports seasons. If you're facing an ordeal like this, don't go without your cushion!

Chronic Coccydynia Requires Expert Help

Most people recover after a period but there are rare instances of chronic coccydynia. If you suspect chronic coccydynia, you will need expert help. Make sure that your healthcare provider understands the seriousness of the problem. Because coccydynia can make it impossible to sit for longer periods of time, ask for help getting your work schedule and work arrangements modified so that you can keep going without making the problem worse.

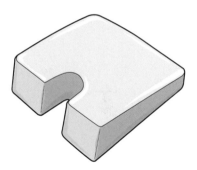

▲ Wedge cushion with coccyx cutout.

Warning! Ask Questions Before Getting an Injection

If your doctor wants to perform an injection, make sure that the person performing the procedure is experienced and has performed this many times in the last year. You can simply ask:

- How many of these injections to the coccyx have you performed in the last year?

- What is your complication rate?

- How long will the effects of the injection last?

- What are the chances that this injection will relieve my pain?

Coccyx injections are usually done with fluoroscopic guidance. This helps avoid injury to delicate structures in the vicinity of the tailbone. Another type of injection that is sometimes used is a ganglion impar block. Although recent studies suggest that this may be an effective treatment, it has traditionally been used in cases where there is a serious structural problem.[3]

PHYSICAL THERAPY IMPROVES BODY MECHANICS

If your doctor tells you that you need physical therapy, you may be wondering what can be done. Several things may be helpful in the setting of coccydynia: pain control will be the first order of business, then focusing on getting the body mechanics right, and some stretching and strengthening may be needed. Rarely, people will need to have manual therapy done in this area. If this is the case, make sure to obtain a specific recommendation for someone with advanced training. Most physical therapists will shy away from the somewhat invasive methods required.

SURGERY IS A RADICAL OPTION

If your doctor recommends surgery, you should consider this step very carefully. Removal of the coccyx is a radical surgery that removes an anchoring point for a complex muscle that is critically important for the functioning of the bowels and the stability of the pelvic floor. The muscles that allow the anus to close properly are connected to the coccyx, and removal of this anchor can produce lasting difficulties with bowel movements. This surgery is usually reserved for situations where there is demonstrated instability of the coccyx that is associated with disabling pain, or in cases where there is a tumor. Be sure to discuss the possible alternatives to surgery and make sure that your doctor paints a very clear picture of what to expect in terms of recuperation and return to daily activities after the surgery. Removal of the coccyx has been reported to have a very high infection rate. This is because the area of the surgery is very close to the bowels, and it is really difficult to keep the area clean. In addition, the recovery is hard to endure, as it is necessary to limit sitting until adequate healing has taken place.

Testing for Coccydynia

The first step in the evaluation of coccydynia is a physician's assessment. Diagnostic testing usually begins with an X-ray, although other imaging tests may follow. Based on the results of the clinical assessment including any test results, your provider will determine if you have a clear structural problem that is causing the pain, or whether treatment will proceed on the basis of a clinical diagnosis.

The examination for coccydynia can consist of a external exam and an internal exam. The external exam will involve the doctor looking at certain structures and palpating various locations in the back and buttock. Some of this will be done to make sure that the problem is not something other than coccydynia. The internal exam for coccydynia is performed for the simple fact that the tailbone in most people is located deep in the buttock, right near the rectum. This is a hard-to-reach location. The internal exam may require the doctor to place a finger inside the rectum and feel for the position and tenderness of the boney tail in this manner.

Some highly specialized physical therapists have been trained to perform manual therapy using this approach. You can imagine that the people who experience problems with muscle spasm in the tailbone area really value people who are willing to learn about and develop the skills needed, but this training is not always appreciated because of the cultural taboos and sensitive nature of these structures.

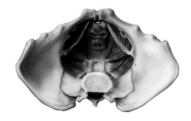

▲ Pelvic floor muscles

The Explanation

Pain emanating from the tail bone is a surprisingly prevalent and troublesome back pain condition. It often is precipitated by a fall in which the person lands suddenly on their bottom. These types of falls are incredibly common. The actual risks that make persistently painful tailbone fracture or injury more or less likely are not known. Childbirth is an important trigger of coccydynia, and not surprisingly, it is estimated to be five times more common in women.

COCCYDYNIA IN CHILDBIRTH

The human tailbone is a small, rudimentary bone that varies from person to person. One important characteristic of each coccyx is the degree to which it is angled or "tucked under." Under ordinary circumstances, having a small tail-remnant that sits more or less tucked under into the rear end of the body is completely without problems. There is one critical juncture however, where having a small bone in this location can be problematic: the moment of childbirth. During the nine months of pregnancy, a developing fetus sits safely inside the abdomen and pelvis of the expectant mother. During these months, hormones gradually work to increase the flexibility and stretchiness of the ligaments that bind the bones of the pelvis to each other. As noted elsewhere in this book, this can cause pain that ranges from mild aching to sharply debilitating if proper steps aren't taken. During labor, the baby descends through the large ring of the pelvis, a process that takes time. Towards the very end of the delivery process, the baby has to slide past the tailbone on its way into the world. Depending on the configuration of the coccyx, the baby will have more or less difficulty passing by this spot.

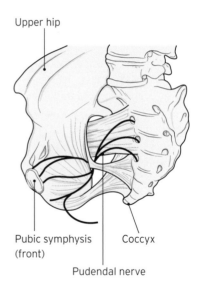

Upper hip

Pubic symphysis (front)

Coccyx

Pudendal nerve

▲ A view of the coccyx seen from inside the pelvis

OTHER PREDISPOSITIONS FOR COCCYDYNIA

Another factor that influences the tendency for pain arising from the tailbone is body weight. A variety of factors that predispose obese people to experience coccydynia; one is a tendency to angle the pelvis in a way that places additional stress on the tailbone when sitting.[4] It has been proposed that plopping down into chairs may be an aggravating factor.

Some people develop coccydynia in association with a minor skeletal malformation of the spine that includes a spicule or sharp spine projecting from the tail end of the coccyx. People with these little spines will typically also have a small dimple in the overlying skin, suggesting that this is the result of a very minor birth defect.[5]

Finally, there are rare instances of tumor or aggressive infection that lead to coccydynia. These conditions require highly specialized treatment and sometimes necessitate consideration of surgical options.

CHAPTER RESOURCES

1. Maigne, J.Y., G. Chatellier, and M.L. Faou, et al. 2006. The treatment of chronic coccydynia with intrarectal manipulation: A randomized controlled study. *Spine* 31 (18): E621-7.

2. Wray, C.C., S. Easom, and J. Hoskinson. 1991. Coccydynia: Aetiology and treatment. *J Bone Joint Surg Br* 73 (2): 335-8.

3. Foye, P.M. "Coccyx Pain," Emedicine. http://emedicine.medscape.com/article/309486-overview. Accessed January 26, 2010.

4. Patel, R., A. Appannagari, and P.G. Whang. 2008. Coccydynia. *Curr Rev Musculoskelet Med* 1 (3-4): 223-26.

5. Foye, P.M. "Coccyx Pain," eMedicine. http://emedicine.medscape.com/article/309486-overview. Accessed January 26, 2010.

6. Cleveland Clinic. Coccydynia, http://my.clevelandclinic.org/disorders/Coccydynia/hic_Coccydynia_Tailbone_Pain.aspx. Accessed January 26, 2010.

7. Foye, P.M. "Coccyx Pain," eMedicine. http://emedicine.medscape.com/article/309486-overview. Accessed January 26, 2010.

Q & A *with Dr. Murinson*

I have coccydynia and feel blue. Is that normal?

Coccydynia can be a very difficult and demoralizing condition to live with. When coccydynia becomes chronic, the impact on daily living is profound. A life in which one cannot sit normally means that regular meals, formal dinners, going to movies, attending cultural events, taking longer car rides, boating, socializing, and many other enjoyable activities are out of the picture until the condition settles down. This can place a substantial strain on family members as well, especially when expectations are high for social interactions or when there are others who may also need care such as young children or aging parents. For this reason, it is important to stay attentive to your state of mind and general mood while living with coccydynia. Feeling down might almost be expected given the challenges, but there is no reason to suffer in silence.[6] There are many medications available that can help improve a depressed mood, and effective non-pharmacological treatments as well. Some of the medications used to treat depressed mood are also known to be effective in reducing pain. If your doctor proposes a medication to help you "feel a little brighter," ask if the medication might also help with the pain. A short list of antidepressants that are known to be pain active includes amitriptyline, desipramine, duloxetine, and venlafaxine. Each of these medications will have a different set of side effects, so a discussion of options with your doctor is needed. If you would prefer to go the non-medication route when addressing depressed mood, ask your doctor if they know of any psychologists or psychiatrists who are well versed in addressing chronic pain. Not all practitioners are tuned in to the needs of patients with persistent pain.

Why is the coccyx so important?

A number of key structures anchor onto the coccyx.[7] These include part of the gluteus muscles (major muscles in the buttock) and muscles that run on either side of the rectum to form part of the floor of the pelvis. Ligaments are present as well. Some of these stabilize the coccyx onto the sacrum, while others run from the coccyx to the ischial tuberosities (sitz bones) on either side. Surgical removal of the coccyx is obviously complicated by the presence of these anchoring support elements. If the coccyx is removed, difficulties with the pelvic floor can follow as the rectum and other pelvic structures begin to sag downward or "prolapse." The consequences can include chronic soiling, incontinence, and increasing pain.

PART 2

Getting Better, Getting Stronger

CHAPTER 13

First Steps for Acute Back Pain

See a practitioner early and often to ensure there is no permanent damage and develop a treatment plan.

the DIANOSIS

> **Are you experiencing serious back pain?**

> **Are you free of any weakness, bowel or bladder incontinence, or numbness?**

Acute management should begin as soon as you develop serious back pain. You will know if the pain is serious by the intensity or degree of pain. Another indicator is if the pain stops you from doing your normal activities. Most doctors, nurses, and other healthcare providers use a 10-point scale to measure pain intensity. If your pain is eight or greater, it is probably serious and you need to seek help. If your pain is less than eight but prevents you from sitting or standing normally, it is serious and you should check in with your doctor. You will probably want to follow the plan in this book.

The primary reason for seeking a diagnosis for serious back pain is to ensure the proper treatment course. You will want to see a doctor, physician's assistant (PA), or nurse practitioner early in the course of back pain to make sure there is no danger to the spinal cord, nerve roots, or other vital structures. Once the dangerous conditions are eliminated as a cause of your back pain (Red Flags for Back Pain), finding a diagnosis may become more challenging, as not all physicians are well trained in the complexities of back structure and function.

RED FLAGS FOR BACK PAIN

If your pain was preceded by a trauma or is associated with weakness or inability to control bowel or bladder functions, you may be dealing with a medical emergency and should seek immediate medical care. Don't do anything else until you see a doctor or qualified medical professional to assess your problem. The Red Flags are:

- Major trauma (car accident, fall from a height)
- Age less than 20 or greater than 50
- History of cancer
- Fever, chills, weight loss
- Recent bacterial infection
- Drug abuse
- Immunosuppression
- Pain that is worse when lying down
- Severe nighttime pain
- New bladder dysfunction (incontinence of urine)
- Numbness over the genitals
- Major or progressive weakness in one or both legs
- Minor trauma, in the setting of low bone density or osteoporosis

Your Clinician Needs to Know:

- Severity of pain (on a 0-10 scale)

- What the pain feels like (sharp, dull, etc.)

- Location of the pain (where it is, where it "goes")

- When the pain started

- What makes it better

- What makes it worse

- Your limitations due to pain

All primary care physicians should be trained to recognize the back pain Red Flags, a term coined by the U.S. Agency for Health Care Policy and Research to aid clinicians in identifying aspects of a patient's medical history or examination that potentially indicate dangerous conditions requiring immediate intervention. These potentially dangerous conditions include spinal fracture, spinal infection, spinal compression, cancer, and nerve root compression. The problem is that even though the red flags were established by a panel of experts and have been around for over a decade, their value in making a diagnosis has not been accurately established, and no one knows for sure how helpful they are as true markers of disease. Suffice it to say that if there is a dangerous condition, you want your doctor to catch it early. The best thing you can do is to provide information about your health as clearly and calmly as possible. You may want to share the Red Flag list with your doctor.

the PRESCRIPTION

There are several very important things that you can do for back pain as soon as it starts:

- Prevent further injury. If you're doing something that has caused you to injure your back, you need to stop doing it.
- Seek medical assessment. You need the help of a medical professional to sort out whether your new back pain could be caused by a serious problem. Once these issues are resolved, you can go forward with treatment and recovery. This step involves finding a physician or care team who will acknowledge the serious nature of your back problem, endeavor to find a diagnosis, address your needs for pain control, connect you with exceptionally good physical therapy, and support your needs for sick leave appropriately.
- Initiate pain control. Early and adequate pain control is vitally important to reduce a person's period of disability, restore normal movement patterns (preventing secondary injury), and reduce the chances of long-term pain. When back pain is serious, it usually requires more than aspirin, ibuprofen, or acetaminophen.

COMMUNICATION IS VITAL TO PAIN CONTROL

It is sometimes hard to explain to a physician or other care provider how badly one's back is hurting. For one thing, many physicians, especially when young, have never experienced serious pain. In our studies, upwards of 30 percent of medical students have never experienced serious physical pain, and many have never considered the impact of pain on the person who is feeling it. On the other hand, older physicians will occasionally become hardened toward the pain of others. Still other physicians hold preconceived notions about back injury and will pigeon-hole patients based on social, economic, gender, or ethnic factors and conclude that the pain is being overstated.

This is critically important because the current medical system relies absolutely on a physician, PA, or nurse to recognize and acknowledge a pain problem before serious medical therapy can be started. Therefore, the first part of beginning pain control is communication.

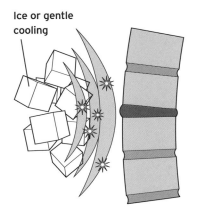

Ice or gentle cooling

▲ Cold therapy helps by reducing local inflammation. Cold works best when used in the first 24 to 48 hours.

Taking Time Off from Work Is No Vacation

One of the biggest problems faced by a person with serious back pain is convincing his or her employer that time off is needed. A concerned and compassionate care provider may be your key to recovery. Many employers require a physician's signature for medical absence from work. But, and this is a critical but, under no circumstances should you take time off from work and not attend physical therapy. If your back pain is serious enough to merit sick leave, you require skilled physical therapy. Sick leave is not vacation, it is time for healing and you must do your part in getting better.

172

The Treatment

If you have to wait for medical assessment, you have some choices to make. You can try using some over-the-counter medications, although serious back pain is often only minimally better with non-prescription medications. Your doctor or nurse will want to know if the pain was relieved by the more common medications, as this will give them potentially valuable diagnostic information about your problem. You should always be thinking about whether massage, acupuncture, ice, warm packs, stretches, rest, or some other non-medication treatment can work with whatever else you're using for pain.

PUT SOME ICE ON IT

One treatment that is often overlooked and under-appreciated is starting with a cold pack. You can almost always help acute back pain with some ice. Why is this? Ice application can help in several important ways. Application of ice or a cold pack will both reduce inflammation after injury and block pain signaling. Often times, patients will give me *that look* when I mention ice packs. That look usually seems to mean "You're kidding. I came to see you so that you could recommend ice packs?" I tell medical students that medical therapy for pain should always, always include non-medication-based treatments in parallel with medications for pain.

HEAT AND TOPICAL AGENTS HELP AFTER 48 HOURS

Although warm therapy is very helpful for chronic low back pain, heating the back may not be very beneficial during the acute phase. Most typically, the first 48 hours after an injury is reserved for cold treatments. After that period, it is often helpful to alternate cold and warm therapies. Warm heat can be delivered in various ways: it is possible to apply warm moist towels, microwave a sachet of buckwheat, use a heating pad, or rub on some medicinal agents that promote warming.

BED REST HELPS WITH SOME BACK PAIN

Proper bed rest is needed for certain types of back pain:

- A disc tear can be excruciatingly painful and is usually more painful when the disc is placed under pressure. Not infrequently, when there is a back injury, a disc is torn. The pain can be quite severe, dull to sharp, and typically located in the center of the back or just to the side. Getting off your feet will decrease the pressure on the disc and help to reduce the pain. An acute disc tear can require a week of bed rest with a gradual increase in activity, but this should only be undertaken with the supervision of a physician experienced in back care. Surprising research showed that the disc has nerve endings; this was not widely appreciated even five years ago. In fact, the outer ring of the spinal disc is richly supplied with pain-sensitive nerve endings.

- A mild disc herniation is not best treated with surgery. Unless you resort to chiropractic manipulation, spine rest can the best way to coax the disc back into place. Bed rest can be combined with gentle traction implemented by a physical therapist, chiropractor, or back-care specialist. Seek the guidance of an experienced rehabilitation specialist regarding the treatment of mild disc herniation with bed rest. Several weeks of graduated activity may be needed with this treatment approach. Be aware that even "mild" disc herniations hurt a lot; studies have shown that the average amount of pain with a herniated disc is eight out of 10!
- A mild flare-up/overdoing it type back pain: often this type of pain is better with a day or two of taking it easy.

BED REST IS NOT HELPFUL FOR MUSCLE PULLS

- A muscle pull is best treated with cold packs, over-the-counter medicines, and avoiding reinjury; bed rest is not ideal, although intermittent rest periods can help.

THE SPINE AT REST

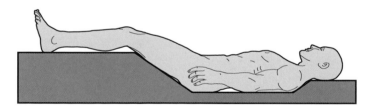

Best position: spine at rest. All possible weight is removed from spine.

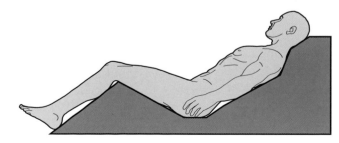

Okay position: spine at partial rest.

Warning! Exercise Caution with Heating Pads

It is important to exercise special care when applying warm therapies. A heating pad should never be applied directly to the skin. It should not be in place for more than 20 minutes, and one should not lay on top of it. It is most prudent not to set the temperature of the heating pad above low. People who have any kind of neuropathy and people who have diabetes, should not use a heating pad unless it is approved by their neurologist. Neuropathy can lead to poor awareness of skin temperatures and damaging burns can result.

Words to Describe the Time Course of Pain

- Explosive onset
- Gradual worsening
- Coming and going for a while
- Ramping up quickly
- Intermittently severe
- Mild and then suddenly worse

The Risks of Pain Control

Medication Reaction

Back Reinjury

Cash Reduction

The Explanation

Pain control is a fundamental need for patients with serious back pain. The benefits of pain control include better quality of life, better prospects for recovery, less disruption of sleep, and a potential reduction in chronic pain.

You must communicate your pain to someone knowledgeable enough to understand the problem and able to order appropriate therapies. This is usually communicated using a 10-point scale where zero is no pain and 10 is the worst pain imaginable. The "pain score" or "pain number" is reproducible and changes quickly when someone obtains relief from pain. The main difficulty with the pain score is that it is subjective, meaning there is no tool or test that will confirm your pain number to someone standing outside of your body. This leads to the next major problem with the pain score: both doctors and nurses will sometimes discount or underestimate a patient's pain score. The obvious consequence is that unperceived pain goes untreated. For this reason, make sure your clinician accurately perceives the seriousness of your back pain as you are feeling it.

For some people, sketching a picture of what the pain onset looked like is helpful.

RISKS WITH PAIN CONTROL

Usually, you will work with your clinician to reduce the risks of pain control. They can be summarized with three R's: Reactions, Reinjury, and Reduced cash.

The first R, for reactions, is the most important. Any and all medications used for pain control carry some side effects, ranging from mild to life threatening. For example, many thousands of people each year suffer gastrointestinal (internal) bleeding as a serious side effect of non-steroidal pain medicines like ibuprofen. It's estimated that more than 16,000 people in the U.S. died from NSAID-induced gastrointestinal bleeding in one year alone! If you take a medicine, be aware of the potential side effects; know the important warning signs and discuss these with your pharmacist. Common medication side effects that may be serious include rashes, excessive fatigue, yellow jaundice, fever, headache, and decreased or discolored urine production. Make sure your doctor, nurse, or care provider speaks with you about the major potential risks of any medication. Write down any questions you have about your prescriptions and call or see your clinician to discuss them. It's a good idea to keep a pain diary and include any medication changes, noting medicines that you take as needed. This is a good place to make notes about which medicines seem to work best and any symptoms you are concerned about.

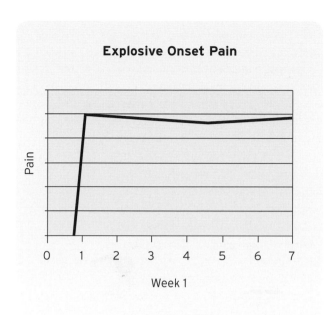

Explosive Onset Pain

Pain

Week 1

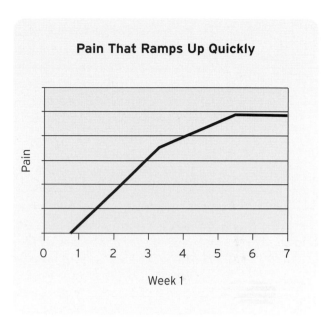

Pain That Ramps Up Quickly

Pain

Week 1

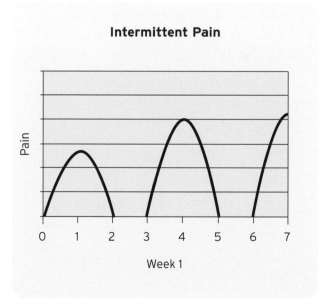

Intermittent Pain

Pain

Week 1

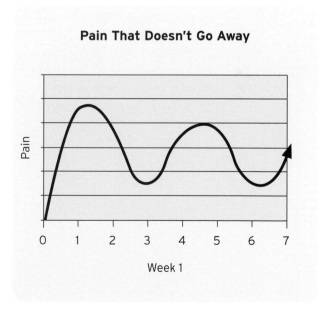

Pain That Doesn't Go Away

Pain

Week 1

The second R is for re-injury, which will hold you back from returning to your life. This book will teach you several techniques to avoid re-injury, ranging from ergonomics and proper back use to core strengthening and positive psychological messaging. Avoiding re-injury seems like the most natural, reasonable goal for someone with serious back pain, and this book is written for just those people seeking a deeper knowledge of the back and spine. Unfortunately, re-injury has become a hot-button issue in the back care industry because fear of re-injury has been identified as slowing the return to work. In reality, you will need to distinguish between reasonable concern arising from experience and unreasonable fear born of anxiety, pressure, and stress. You will have to make conscious decisions in order to protect your back from this day forward; you will need to think about how to bend, how to lift, when not to move heavy objects, when to take rest breaks and how to select and modify your shoes. In the short run, having a little pain to warn you away from back-endangering activities can be helpful.

The third R is not so much a risk as a reality. All treatments cost money; the objective is to find a highly effective treatment for the lowest cost. Ask your doctor to consider generic alternatives, especially if your insurance will not cover the cost of your medication. It's okay to let your doctor know if you are having trouble paying for medicines and to discuss how your treatment can include lower-cost options. Keep in contact with your insurance company about the range of treatments that may be needed for your back. Bear in mind that not treating a back injury will also have a cost, and you will need to balance the cost of treatment with the cost of continued pain. A major message of this book is that the consistent application of non-drug therapies such as cold, heat, ergonomic-positioning, physical therapy, and clinical psychological techniques will help to reduce dependence on medications and potentially make the medications you take more effective against your pain.

Q & A *with Dr. Murinson*

I injured my back, but it wasn't until hours later that it began to hurt. Why is that?

At first it may be hard to believe that you have been hurt, especially if you are otherwise busy, healthy, and active. Accidents occur unexpectedly and are a frequent cause of back pain. It's easy to understand that shock and surprise can delay people from recognizing the seriousness of a problem. Sometimes, the precipitating back injury seems inexplicably minor compared to the pain that follows, and this will delay problem recognition. And although back pain can start almost immediately with accidental injury, it often takes several hours for the pain to set in, and sometimes even longer. Days can pass before pain peaks. Delayed pain is common for people that are injured under "battlefield" conditions, reflecting physiological factors like the release of stress hormones. Delayed pain can happen when someone is focusing intently on completing a task, reflecting psychological factors such as attention and pain distraction. Delayed pain can occur in performance-related settings where all eyes are on you and a premium is paid for "going on with the show." Finally, delayed pain may be due to the nature of the injury and the underlying disease process at work (pathophysiological factors) such as delayed swelling or inflammation.

My pain changes from day to day. How can I communicate that on a pain scale?

One very valuable tool for communicating with your doctors and care providers about your pain is the pain diary or pain calendar. It can be as simple as jotting a single pain score on a wall calendar each day, or as elaborate as a keeping a detailed journal of each day's experiences. With the basic pain tally each day, it is very easy for your doctor to tell how things are going at a glance. It will make it possible to gauge whether a new therapy is working and alternatively, can help you assess your progress as you return to work or school. Also, people gain a sense of control over their pain simply by writing it down. Gaining control over your pain and getting your life back is the ultimate goal of treatment for back pain.

CHAPTER 14

Early Exercises for Managing Back Pain

With Lina Mezei, certified yoga instructor. Gentle yoga can offer significant pain relief and increase mobility.

the PRESCRIPTION

 ## Warning! Easy Does It

Never push yourself to the point of pain. Yoga for back pain is not supposed to be strenuous; rather, it is meant to be restorative and healing.

Warning! Check with Your Doctor

Be sure to check with your doctor for specific warnings against any of the exercises described in this chapter before beginning.

If you are in the early stages of recovering from back pain and you are able to sit for 20 minutes, stand up from a chair without wincing, and tie your own shoes, these early exercises for acute back pain may be right for you.

It's time to learn about yoga, a system of poses, breathing, and thoughtful meditation that has been used for thousands of years to promote health. You can take a gentle yoga class, borrow books from the library, get a yoga DVD, or talk it over with a knowledgeable friend.

- Your first yoga practice should be very gentle and well within your comfort zone. If you feel pain, it is time to backtrack and get more guidance. There is an excellent DVD produced by *Yoga Journal* called *Yoga for Your Pregnancy*. While you may not be pregnant, you can imagine that yoga for pregnancy is very, very gentle. This is where you want to begin.
- The yoga exercises in this chapter were adapted from standard yoga postures. They reflect the recommendations for improved core stability and gentle stretching.

Where to Practice Yoga

Yoga is primarily practiced on a yoga mat in a warm room, which aids in making your muscles more loose and flexible. For extra padding, you may want to place your yoga mat on a carpeted surface. Throughout all of the yoga poses, be conscious of your breathing. If, while in a posture, your breath becomes labored, it means you need to back off a bit. It is important that you listen to your body and modify the extent of poses and stretches as you see fit.

The Treatment

The best way to start is to practice yoga breathing: refreshing breaths that reach deep into the lower abdomen. This is sometimes more challenging for women, as many women have learned over time to breath with the chest and not as much with the abdomen. Babies breathe with the abdomen; think about the gentle rise and fall of the belly with each breath.

In yoga, we use a technique called Ujjayi breathing, which translates into victorious breathing. Breathing should be completely unrestricted, each inhalation slow and expansive. As you practice controlling your breathing so it is longer and stronger, you should eventually be able to feel your breath deep inside your belly. This type of deep belly breathing requires some practice; each exhale should be steady and completely emptying.

There are two exercises one can do to practice Ujjayi breathing. One method is to take a deep, full inhalation and exhale as if you were fogging up a car window on a cold day. Another method is to whisper the word "home." While whispering, draw out each sound of the word so that it takes roughly three to five seconds for you to complete each whisper. If done properly, you should feel a slight constriction of air in the back of the throat and the exhale should be very audible. These breathing exercises can also increase lung capacity and stamina for performing your yoga sequences. Additionally, practicing controlled yogic breath work is attributed to creating balance within the autonomic nervous system and fostering physical and mental tranquility.[1, 2] Different yogic traditions place varying degrees of emphasis on control of the breath.[3] Although many advocate breathing in through the nose and out through the mouth, it is possible to breath in and out through the nose; if breathing in through the nose feels too restrictive, to breath in and out through the mouth.

LIE DOWN FOR BASIC VINYASA

Yoga is structured into specific sequences called *vinyasas*, which translates into "flowing movement." Your yoga practice should move with fluidity, each pose flowing into the next in correlation with your breathing to make each posture more restorative and beneficial. The goals of this basic vinyasa are to warm up, gain focus, concentrate on breathing, stretch, and awaken the spine.

1. Lying down *Tadasana* (Mountain Pose) will prepare and provide focus for your yoga sequence. This pose will get you acquainted with your yoga mat as well. Lay your body face-up on the mat. Adjust yourself so that your body experiences maximum contact with the mat. This may require you to move the flesh around your sitz bones in order to make better contact. Gently rock your spine side to side and up and down until you feel an imprint in the mat. Keep legs together and your feet flexed as though you are standing on an imaginary floor. Your arms should be placed next to your sides, hands open with your palms touching your thighs or in prayer at the center of your chest. Become aware of your body as you pull your belly in towards your spine. There should be no tension in this pose, so make sure your shoulders are down away from the ears and relaxed. Concentrate on alignment while breathing. Imagine you are as steady and strong as a mountain. As you begin, you may need a small support under the head and a small bolster under the knees. By the end of the early back pain phase, your goal is to be able to lie flat.

2. Transition from Mountain Pose to lying down *Vrksasana* (Tree Pose). Vrksasana is a nice hip-opening posture that will also help to release tension in the pelvis. Simply bring up one leg and place the sole of the foot against the inner thigh. If this is difficult, place the foot firmly on the inner shin. Adjust yourself so that the pelvis and hips are in a neutral/straight position, and not jutting out toward the side that your foot is pressing on. For complete engagement, flex the foot of your outstretched leg. Press your hands together in a prayer position in the center of the chest. For an even greater stretch, lift your arms over your head, interlace your fingers, and turn your hands so that the palms face away from your head. Relax, take a few deep breaths, and repeat with the other leg.

A precursor to Bandhasana ▶
(Bridge Pose)

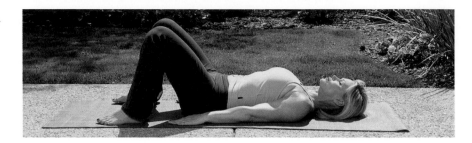

3. Now that your pelvis has been stabilized, practice a precursor to *Setu Bandhasana* (Bridge Pose). In this early phase, the posture will be presented as pre-bridge pelvic tilts. While laying flat on your back, bend your knees and walk your heels toward your buttocks. Your feet should be flat on the mat and a hip-width apart. Place your fingertips toward the heels while lengthening your neck and pressing the lower back into the mat. Press all four corners of the feet firmly into the mat. As you exhale, engage your abdominal muscles and buttocks. Begin to tilt your pelvis, making your tailbone curl up as your whole lower back presses into the mat. The small of your lower back should feel completely flat. Hold here for three breaths and slowly release on an exhale. Repeat these movements three to five more times while moving with your breath. This posture aids in toning and relieving pressure in the lower spine.

4. Roll over onto the belly to prepare for a modified *Ardha Salabhasana* (Half Locust Pose). This variation is the least difficult locust posture, yet it is capable of relieving much tension in the lower back.[4] Lie flat, placing your palms face down alongside the hips, or tucked underneath the thighs. Push firmly down on the hands, pelvis, and pubic bone as you gently inhale and raise the right leg upward two to four inches off of the mat. Make sure the raised leg is straight and the toes are pointing directly behind your body. Exhale as you slowly lower your right leg back down to the mat. Repeat three to five more times, then switch to the left leg. This posture activates the extensor muscles along the spine, namely the erector spinae and mutifidus muscles.

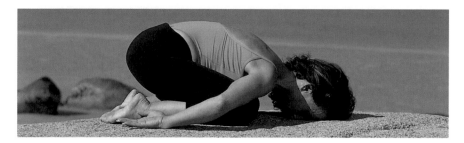

◀ Balasana (Child's Pose)

5. A wonderful counter-stretch to *Ardha Salabhasana*, which is a back extension exercise, is a gentle spinal flexion such as supported *Balasana* (Child's Pose). You will need a pillow for the supported version. Begin by getting onto your knees, resting the tops of the feet flat on the mat, and positioning them directly behind the buttocks. The knees splay out toward the front corners of the mat. Place the pillow comfortably underneath your belly and chest. Take a deep breath in, and on your exhale, slowly begin to lower your belly, chest, and forehead down toward the mat, allowing your heart to sink into the pillow. Place your arms outstretched in front of you with your palms facing down on the mat. Allow the rest of your body to sink into the floor and begin to melt away into your mat. Relax in this pose while taking five to ten deep, restorative breaths.

6. After releasing *Balasana*, move the pillow away and gently roll over onto your back to prepare for the next posture, a modified *Ardha Apanasana* (Half Wind-Relieving Posture). Apanasana is a flexion posture designed to open your hips and to stabilize your pelvis and lower back. While laying flat on your back, allow the whole spine to press down into the mat. Raise the right knee up and in toward the chest on an inhale. If strain is caused by trying to bring your knee to the chest, just lift your leg so that your thigh and knee are directly above your hip and your calf is at a 90-degree angle from your thigh with your foot flexed. On each long inhalation, allow the belly to expand. On each long exhalation, continue to pull the knee closer toward your chest. On your third breath, gently glide the knee toward the opposite side so that the knee cap is pointing in the direction of the left shoulder. Hold your leg here for three breaths. Switch legs by releasing and extending your right leg as you bring your left knee up toward your chest and repeat the sequence.

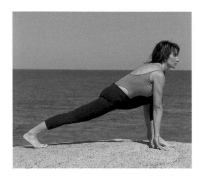

▲ A modified Virabhandrasana (Warrior Pose) forward lunge with hands providing balance and support

STANDING POSES IN BASIC VINYASA

1. Prepare for a modified *Virabhandrasana* (Warrior Pose) by bringing yourself to a standing position, in which your body is upright and you are resting lightly on your feet. It is a good idea to place your mat over carpet and next to a wall in case you need to reach out for stability. Place your right foot about two feet in front of your body, and lean forward, aligning the right knee directly over the heel. As you lean forward on the right leg, try to keep the heel of the left foot on the ground as you stretch your calf and hip muscles. As you are more comfortable in this position and would like to experience a more intense stretch, move your right foot further forward, working towards a distance of three feet between your feet. Remain in this gentle lunge position as you visualize reaching upward through the crown of your head for five to eight breaths. Keep your shoulders down back so that they are not scrunching up towards the ears, with your hands by your sides. After three to five breaths, return to your original standing position and switch to stretch your left leg. It is beneficial to incorporate postures that stretch the hip flexors, as low back pain and lumbar lordosis are often exacerbated by tightness in these muscles.[5]

   Once you are comfortable with the supported forward lunge, you can progress to a Virabhadrasana I (Warrior I Pose) by first bringing your torso into an upright position. Breathing in through your nose, raise your arms straight up and reach for the ceiling, framing your ears with your forearms. Engage your left leg by lifting up on the quadriceps and left kneecap. Tuck your tailbone, suck your belly in toward your spine, and continue reaching up with your fingertips. Make sure your shoulders are down and back as you hold Warrior I pose. After five breaths, bring your left foot forward to prepare for stretching on the other side.

2. Now that your quadriceps and hips have been stretched, it is time to engage your leg and core muscles in a wall-assisted *Utkatasana* (Fierce Pose). It has been recognized in back pain sufferers that weakness in core musculature creates a biomechanical deficit.[6] It is crucial to strengthen the core, which helps to stabilize the spine, which in turn helps to relieve pain. To start, walk over to the nearest flat wall. Position your body so that your buttocks are resting comfortably against the wall. Your feet should be out in front of you so that your heels are approximately a foot (30 cm) or so away from the wall. Stand with the feet hip-width distance apart as you begin to slide your buttocks down the wall. You should appear to be sitting in a chair but leaning forward a bit. Raise your arms up overhead, framing your ears with your forearms. Be mindful that there is

no tension in the shoulders, as the shoulder blades should be down and back. Make sure that your tailbone is tucked under and that you are sucking your belly in towards your spine. Concentrate on the breath as you reach for the ceiling on every inhale and sink a bit lower and deeper on every exhale. Hold for five breaths. As an alternative to this pose, it is possible to substitute a wall slide until the back is strong enough for you to lean forward away from the wall.

3. Turn so that the front of your body is facing toward a support such as a wall to prepare for a modified *Adho Mukha Svanasana* (Downward-Facing Dog Pose). Stand facing the wall with your arms outstretched at shoulder width. Press the palms flat against the wall at chest level. You should be standing with your feet apart at hip-width distance. While firmly pressing both hands into the wall, slowly begin to walk your feet back. Your shoulder blades should be down, away from the ears. Begin to feel a huge opening in your shoulders and spine as you allow your head and chest to sink down past your arms. Your feet should be planted firmly into the ground with your legs straight or with a slight bend in the knees. Hold here for eight long, restorative breaths. This modified version of Downward-Facing Dog provides a multitude of benefits including stretching most of the long muscles of the body. This pose also provides active lengthening of the erector spinae and latismus dorsi muscles. Lengthening the back extensor muscles greatly reduces low back compression.

4. While still facing the wall, prepare for a variation on a primer pose for *Natarajasana* (Dancer). Stand arm's-length away from the wall and place your right palm flat against it at shoulder height. Kick your right leg behind your body. Bend the knee to bring the heel of the right foot close to the right buttock. Take the left hand and reach back and around to grab the inside of the right arch. Actively lift that right foot with your left hand to feel a wonderful opening in the quadriceps and iliopsoas muscles. Repeat on the left side.

5. Now that the quadriceps and iliopsoas muscles have been stretched, it is time for a gentle back extension posture, *Anuvittasana* (Standing Backbend). Stand in *Tadasana*, reaching the crown of the head toward the ceiling while lifting the chest and ribcage. Bring the palms of the hands to the lower back, right above the buttocks. As you exhale, drop the head slightly back and press your hips and thighs forward. Bring your gaze upward. On your fifth breath, slowly inhale the head back to vertical followed by the rest of the body.

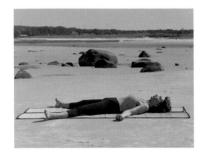

▲ Savasana (Corpse Pose)

6. One final back flexion exercise that releases the entire spinal column is a seated *Uttanasana* (Forward Fold/Ragdoll). Sit in a chair and place your feet firmly on the ground. Take a big inhalation as you raise your arms up overhead, creating length along the entire spine. Sustain that length by reaching out and forward with your arms as you begin to flex at your hips to lower your belly onto your thighs. Your arms should hang loose, with one arm at the side of each shin. Let the head hang heavy over your knees as you begin to release all tension in the neck. During the early phase after back pain, it is better to lean forward into a bolster.

7. Always end your yoga practice with five or ten minutes of deep breathing meditation in *Savasana* (Corpse Pose). A bolster under the knees and shins is a good prop to incorporate during this early phase, as it will assist in relieving tension in the low back. This is the total relaxation pose, which for many is the most difficult pose to master. While laying flat on your back, close your eyes, spread your legs about hips-width apart, and place your arms out by your sides with the palms facing up toward the ceiling. Try to loosen all the muscles in your face and body and begin to take slow, steady, deep inhalations and exhalations through your nose and mouth. Be still, clear your mind, and visualize yourself as being weightless. Do not underestimate the power of relaxation for back pain relief. General muscle tightness, tension, and spasms resulting from life's daily stresses contribute to back pain.[7]

Practice these poses daily. For best results, try for multiple times throughout the day. After a few weeks of persistent and steady practice, you should be ready to move on to some more restorative and strengthening poses.[8,9]

The Explanation

Yoga is a phenomenal way to get in touch with your body. As you practice yoga, you will begin to notice improvements in breathing, body awareness, posture, mobility, stability, and agility. Many of the physical therapy exercises that are used today have direct correlates in the centuries-old yoga poses described here.

CHAPTER RESOURCES

1. Brown, R.P. and P.L. Gerbarg. 2009. Yoga Breathing, Meditation, and Longevity. Longevity, Regeneration, and Optimal Health. *Ann. N.Y. Acad. Sci.* 1172:54-62.

2. Nayak, N.N. and K. Shankar. 2004. *Yoga: A Therapeutic Approach. Physical Medicine and Rehabilitation Clinics of North America* 15: 783-798.

3. McCall, T. *Yoga as Medicine: The Yogic Prescription for Health and Healing.* Bantam Books, New York, 2007.

4. Coulter, D.H. *Anatomy of Hatha Yoga: A Manuel for Students, Teachers, and Practitioners.* Honesdale, PA: Body and Breath, 2001.

5. Borg-Olivier, S. and B. Machliss. "Yoga for Low-Back Pain: Simple Yoga Stretches And Exercises Can Help Alleviate The Highest Cause Of Sick Leave, Say Physiotherapists Simon Borg-Olivier and Bianca Machliss." *Complementary Medicine Journal*, November/December 2005.

6. Sorosky, S., S. Stilp, and V. Akuthota. 2008. Yoga and pilates in the management of low back. *Curr Rev Musculoskeletal Med* 1: 39-47.

7. Borg-Olivier, S. and B. Machliss. "Yoga for Low-Back Pain: Simple Yoga Stretches And Exercises Can Help Alleviate The Highest Cause Of Sick Leave, Say Physiotherapists Simon Borg-Olivier and Bianca Machliss." *Complementary Medicine Journal*, November/December 2005.

8. Sherman, K.J., D.C. Cherkin, J. Erro, D.L. Miglioretti, and R.A. Deyo. 2005. Comparing yoga, exercise, and a self-care book for chronic low back pain: A randomized, controlled trial. *Annals of Internal Medicine* 143 (12): 849-56.

9. Williams, K. A., et al. 2005. Effect of Iyengar yoga therapy for chronic low back pain. *Pain* 115 (1-2): 107-17.

CHAPTER 15

Shaping Your Own Recovery

Consistent self-care is just as important as medical intervention

the DIAGNOSIS

> **Have you had back pain for longer that you ever thought you would?**

> **Have you been trying everything the doctors tell you without good results?**

> **Are you unsure that anyone really understands what's happening with your back?**

Back pain is the most common pain problem in the U.S. today. It is the number-one cause of work-related disability and a huge expense in terms of doctor visits, over-the-counter and prescription medications, physical therapy treatments, and surgical procedures. For all this investment of time, effort, and money, we have little positive to show. Most of the therapies that we doctors have are at best partially effective. The current standards for pain treatments are that they have to reduce pain by 50 percent. Usually by the time someone has had back pain for several months, there's a chance that whatever we do to make it better will only help a little bit.

This book is written to be a new solution to back pain, and this chapter is the key element. All the other chapters of this book are designed to bring together the best that medicine and science has to offer about the back and to put this information into your hands. But this chapter asks the question: "What are you going to do to make your back pain better?" You must be the captain of your own ship. You are an adult and have a responsibility to yourself and your close ones to take command of your health.

In truth, whatever positive steps you take will have a greater cumulative impact than all the medical interventions out there. This is true for almost all the problems that are not clearly medical emergencies. Take smoking, for example. If all the smokers in the country were to stop smoking, most of our highly trained cardiologists would be sitting around waiting for the next patient to show up. We would probably need a third fewer hospital beds and medical equipment makers would have a drastic drop in demand. The same applies for obesity, excessive alcohol consumption, and most other long-term health problems. Honestly, some people have a genetic predisposition to certain problems. But each person who makes peace with their back has come to a certain point: the place where outside solutions aren't working anymore and a new, custom-tailored plan of action is born. If you're not there yet, I hope you can start to take small steps and look carefully for improvement. Ask the questions: "What will I do for my back today?" followed by "What can I do better?", "What can I learn?" "Is there something new that I haven't tried yet for my back?", and "Who can teach me?"

If you are ready to be the master of your back's destiny, read on!

the PRESCRIPTION

Rest Works Wonders

While you are living with back pain, start any task early and take breaks to lie down. Putting the back to rest and taking some deep breaths will make a world of difference. It is widely recognized among experienced pain practitioners that a period of overdoing it is inevitably followed by a period of increased pain; this is sometimes referred to as the pain-rest cycle.[1]

- Identify healthcare professionals and treatments that work for you.
- Advocate for your own health needs. Speak openly with your doctor and others about your back pain and how treatments are working. A pain calendar or journal is a great way to keep track of your progress and pitfalls.
- Pace yourself. Don't let others intimidate you into pushing too hard. Overdoing it while your back is getting better is a mistake and may lead to long-term problems.
- Use all therapies with proper care. Many of the treatments for back pain have unintended side effects, including physical therapy. Be well informed and speak up if something's not right.
- Acknowledge that pain probably has physical and psychological components.
- Avoid or opt out of activities that repeatedly make your back pain worse. At one end of the spectrum, this means not going on a ski trip; at the other end, a career change may be the most important life change you can make.
- Use pain relievers judiciously. There is such a thing as too much and, believe it or not, too little. Severe pain early after an injury can actually lead to chronic pain.
- Visualize your life without back pain. You can do this as a form of meditation or write some affirmations and paste them to your mirror.
- Let people know how you're doing. You will find that all the caring you've shared with others over the years will come back to you.
- Learn about your back and develop your own strategies for a back-healthy lifestyle. Build a personalized plan of exercise, movement, medication, and meditation.

The Treatment

If your recovery is difficult and takes longer than initially expected, you may need to switch therapists or doctors. It's fair to say to someone, "I appreciate that you've brought me this far and thank you," and move on for a fresh perspective.

ALTERNATIVE TREATMENTS ALSO CARRY RISKS

The prescribed medications available in the U.S. are subject to careful scrutiny before approval for use and are subsequently manufactured with stringent standards. Despite this, problems still arise. In stark contrast, dietary supplements are manufactured under loosely regulated conditions and are completely unproven in terms of providing a health benefit. The essential standard for a dietary supplement is that it must not be harmful and that any claims made must be backed up by scientific studies. However, the safety of dietary supplements is not tested before they are brought to market. As the supplements are sold, the FDA monitors for harmful effects and will compel the withdrawal of a product that proves to be unsafe.[2] If you take a dietary supplement, you are part of a real-time social experiment that may result in people like you suffering harm. One example of a potentially harmful dietary supplement is vitamin B_6. When B_6 is taken at mega-vitamin levels, it causes painful neuropathy that may take months to recover from.

Chiropractic manipulation can cause strokes when performed with excessive vigor in the neck region. Acupuncture can be hazardous if the practitioner is not reputable and experienced. Many of the conventional treatments for back pain, including lumbar epidural steroid injections, radiofrequency ablation, surgery, and medications can all be harmful if not used with appropriate caution and care.

PAIN IS STRONGLY IMPACTED BY STRESS

For most people, pain is a complex mixture of physical and psychological components.

This does not mean the problem is in your head. It means that stress levels have a big impact on the perception and experience of pain. I've had plenty of patients with seriously painful nerve problems who find that pain is better during vacation. This doesn't mean that the pain is made up; it means that coping mechanisms may not be functioning as well under everyday circumstances and that with proper steps, some of the pain relief they experience while on vacation could be brought to bear in "real-time."

LEARN MORE ABOUT PAIN RELIEVERS

Many pain relievers can be used for the treatment of back pain: classic NSAIDs, acetaminophen, and opioids; pain-active antidepressants including tricyclics and newer serotonin-norepinephrine reuptake inhibitors; anticonvulsants such as the

Warning! Allergic Reactions Demand Immediate Response

If you think you are having a medication allergy, it is best to get help immediately. Some medications, especially muscle relaxants, anticonvulsants, and antidepressants can have serious effects with abrupt withdrawal. If you stop a prescribed medicine suddenly, you need to contact your doctor or the on-call physician about this.

The Benefits of Aerobic Exercise

- Reduced stress
- Greater ease in accomplishing everyday tasks
- Pain relief
- Improved pain tolerance
- Better mental functioning
- Aids weight control and weight loss

newer gabapentin and pregabalin as well as older ones such as carbamazepine; and neuro-modulating agents that are sometimes injected or used locally, including lidocaine and methylprednisolone acetate (Depomedrol). Each medication within a class has slightly different side effects and properties of action: how long it stays in the system, whether it is metabolized by kidney or liver, and how it interacts with other medications. The cost, too, can influence whether it is right or not.

One other medication option is the use of topical medications. Lidocaine is now available in a patch placed right over the painful area. A surprising number of people experience relief from this treatment. Also, some formulations of NSAIDs come in topical creams that are rubbed into the body. The opioid medication fentanyl is available as a prescription patch. This does not work by local action, but rather delivers the medication in a way that affects the entire body.

The specifics of your back problem will determine which medications might be right for you. If there is a nerve pain component to your back pain (zinging, burning, or shock-like pains), you may need to take prescription medication. Your doctor can provide instructions for a special compounding pharmacy to make customized medications. There are many options, so don't give up hope of getting relief.

DON'T LET JOB WORRIES RUIN YOUR LIFE

If you are able to work while your back recovers, great. If you need time to focus on getting better, you're going to have to ask. But don't attempt to game the system and use this time to engage in activities that will interfere with your recovery. Ask your care provider to support your need for time off during the acute phase and recovery. You'll need to do your part by attending physical therapy, keeping good records, and taking medications appropriately.

If you are prone to back pain with prolonged sitting, see if you can do your job while standing up from time to time. It might be possible to make phone calls while standing or get an adapted workstation that allows position changes. You may even need to change jobs to accommodate your physical constraints. This is the most difficult decision that I've seen patients make, but sometimes a necessary choice, and the best one in terms of correcting a chronic pain problem.

DEVELOP AN EXERCISE AND RECOVERY PLAN THAT WORKS FOR YOU

Getting back to an improved state of health is the best defense against back pain. Perhaps the most distinctive feature of a healthy lifestyle is exercise. Simply put, the value of getting aerobic exercise three times a week cannot be overstated. Choosing an exercise that you find enjoyable and rewarding, and getting into the habit of breaking a sweat three times weekly is the single best thing you can do to prevent a recurrence of back pain. Frequent exercise will make everything else you do easier; it will reduce overall stress, increase your pain tolerance, reduce your residual pain, and improve your chances of staying mentally sharp for years to come. Although you should check with your doctor before starting a new exercise routine, push ahead until you get that clearance and then go!

The Explanation

Increasingly, medical researchers are finding that people with certain personality features are more likely to get better from an injury. One of the essential elements of doing well after a back problem is a sense of self-efficacy, a belief that you have the power to make positive decisions. The effects of self-efficacy were recognized several decades ago in the nursing research literature where a related concept called the *internal locus of control* was described. In this, a person believes that they are responsible for events and the outcomes of their experiences. People without this feel that others have control over them. People with a good internal locus of control are generally healthier and have better health outcomes.[3, 4] This is being echoed in the current pain literature, which finds that people with better self-efficacy survive and even go on to thrive, despite adverse events.[5]

Like all doctors with back pain patients, I've had people come in saying "Doc, I'll do anything you tell me." Most often, this is the patient who refuses to change anything in response to our conversations. They refuse to start physical therapy because they've tried that before and it didn't work; they refuse to try a new medicine because their primary care doctor (friend, neighbor) didn't approve; they refuse to start exercising because they just don't have the time. The simple fact is this patient is not ready to get better. They are trapped in a cycle of believing that someone somewhere is going to solve their problem without any effort from them. This won't happen. No one, not even your surgeon, is going to have the magic solution to fix all back pain. You're going to need answers, but in reality, the answer is: you.

Ask for Help

Friends and family are especially important as you go through an experience of serious back pain. Especially if you have small children or pets, the lifting and bending tasks are endless. Just finding someone who can lift a child into the car can be a wonderful act of kindness. If they are open to being helpful, don't be embarrassed to arrange for help again.

Exceptional Resources for Shaping Your Own Recovery

Overall
Managing Chronic Pain Workbook by John D. Otis

7 Minutes of Magic by Lee Holden

Exercise-focused
Mindfulness Yoga by Frank J. Boccia

Banish Your Back Pain the Pilates Way by Anne Shelby

Taking care of your body
The Trigger Point Therapy Workbook by Clair Davies

Move into Life by Anat Baniel

CHAPTER RESOURCES

1. Otis, J.D. *Managing Chronic Pain*. New York: Oxford University Press, 2007.

2. NCCAM. "Using Dietary Supplements Wisely," http://nccam.nih.gov/health/supplements/wiseuse.htm. Accessed February 12, 2010.

3. Waldron, B., et al. 2010. Health locus of control and attributions of cause and blame in adjustment to spinal cord injury. *Spinal Cord* [Epub].

4. Nyland, J., B. Cottrell, K. Harreld, and D.N. Caborn. 2006. Self-reported outcomes after anterior cruciate ligament reconstruction. *Arthroscopy* 22 (11): 1225-32.

5. Foster, N.E., et al. 2009. Distinctiveness of psychological obstacles to recovery in low-back pain patients in primary care. *Pain* [Epub].

CHAPTER 16

Ergonomics

Design your home and work environment for optimal back health

Warning! Use Proper Technique

Part of taking back your back is changing how you do those tasks that are especially hard on the back. You must use proper technique to resume certain activities.

Did You Know?

The study of ergonomics extends back in time to the ancient Romans and perhaps beyond. Bernardo Rammazini (1633-1714), however, is recognized as the founder of occupational medicine.[1] His landmark work, translated into English as *A Treatise on the Diseases of Tradesmen*, contained many chapters devoted to the maladies of a particular occupation. Of those who sit, he noted "All sedentary workers...are a bad color, and in poor condition...for when the body is not kept moving, the blood becomes tainted, its waste matter lodges in the skin, and the condition of the whole body deteriorates."[2]

What Is Ergonomics?

Ergonomics is a "new" word created in the late 1940s by a British scientist interested in designing better work environments. Hywell Murrell was a chemist by training; one wonders how he developed an interest in work environments, but clearly the process of studying how humans function best and how to make their environments more productive and less pain-provoking was a revolutionary idea.

There are some basic principles of ergonomics that will allow you to maximize your back health. Especially if you sit at a desk or work on the computer for much of the day, there are some simple things that you can do to ease pressure on the spine. Reducing spine pressure is critical for speeding recovery from back injury and increasing your quality of life in the long term. Not only discs but ligaments, muscles, and joints will respond negatively to excess pressures and strains. There are special ergonomic considerations that apply to specific types of back problems.

There are a dozen easy things you can do to preserve your back at work if you feel as though you're working hard to get simple tasks accomplished or as though your enviornment is working against you:

When Sitting:
1. Get a lumbar cushion for your chair and lean back into it. By leaning back you can transfer the weight of your upper body onto the chair and reduce the pounds of pressure on the discs and other back structures.
2. Adjust the height of your chair so that your feet rest lightly on the ground. A healthy sitting stance depends on getting your pelvis into neutral. This can only happen if your feet are able to provide support and your legs are not sloping up or down. If you cannot get a chair that is the proper height, consider carrying a lightweight footrest.
3. Sit directly in front of your task area, sitting square to the work surface. Symmetry is an essential element of succeeding against back pain every day. Sit up straight whenever possible.

When Standing:

4. Wear shoes that have cushioned insoles. This will reduce the impact each step has on the spine, knees, and hips. Especially if you spend a lot of time walking over hard floors, you should strive for the best footwear possible. You can sometimes improve less expensive shoes by adding an athletic or high-density heel cushion or full foot support.

5. As you stand, tighten your abdominal muscles and try to maintain a pelvic neutral position. Visualize how a dancer would stand and draw yourself up tall. Hold this as long as possible and then relax with some deep, cleansing breaths.

6. If you must stand for a long period of time, a firm rubber floor mat will help relieve pressure on your back and reduce fatigue and pain.

7. Stand as if your head is floating off of your shoulders, lifted by a helium balloon. This approach comes from the Alexander Technique. It is a great tension reliever. Stand as if your head is being gently lifted up and forward by a string; this will immediately improve your posture (and may even brighten your outlook).

8. Hold your shoulders back and take deep abdominal breaths through the nose. Shift your weight and intermittently contract key posture muscles like the abdominals and the muscles of the buttock. Stretch a little as you bend from side to side and pull your shoulder blades together.

When Lifting:

9. If you must carry a load, make it light and put it into a backpack worn on both shoulders. Better yet, consider a rolling cart or rolling bag. Be careful not to get hurt when lifting the bag or cart into a car or over an obstacle.

10. When lifting, never bend forward or to the side with your back bent. To pick up objects safely, you must bend at the knees and keep your bottom low; lift with the legs. You won't be ready to lift again until you've 1) strengthened your buttock and thigh muscles; and 2) stretched out your calf muscles to stabilize the heel on the ground.

11. Bend your knees and tighten your abdominals as much as possible when lifting or shoveling. You shouldn't start lifting or shoveling until your recovery phase is completed and you feel strong and pain-free for several months. When you are back to good health, use proper technique to avoid new back problems. Set a realistic goal for yourself like being able to do 20 crunches before pitching in with a shoveling or lifting project.

12. Take a break every hour and put the back to rest two or more times a day, once a day if recovery is complete. It is important to stretch and move about, especially if you are sitting in a chair much of the day. Your legs, eyes, neck, lungs, and heart will also benefit.

The Treatment

The amount of pressure on the spinal discs is lowest when we are lying down. The pressure increases with standing and sitting. In the sitting position, the amount of pressure depends on how much weight is coming downwards on the spine. So when people are in acute disc pain, they may grab the arms of a chair as they lower themselves gently down into the seat. This reduces the transient pressure peak that occurs at the moment we sit but does not change the pressure once sitting.

LEAN BACK WHEN SITTING

When sitting is very painful, it is best to minimize the time spent sitting. Once sitting becomes possible again, it is beneficial to lean back. It has been shown that by leaning back, we can transfer the weight of the upper body onto the chair back. By leaning back even 10 degrees from the vertical, it is possible to reduce disc pressures by a substantial amount. How much is 10 degrees? Think of the minute hand of a clock at three minutes past the hour; that is nine degrees off the vertical. Sounds simple, right? Try it and see if it will work for you.

LUMBAR CUSHIONS BRACE THE SPINE

A lumbar cushion will help to place the spine in a protective curvature and transfer weight off of your back and onto the chair. There are a number of different lumbar cushions, and what feels good for you early after an injury may not be right for you later. Your physical therapist may be able to supply a lumbar roll or McKenzie roll, or may be able to direct you to good resources for them. You may also want to ask your doctor to prescribe one.

A HEADSET MAKES SENSE

Try getting a telephone headset if you don't have one already. The ability to talk without cradling a phone on your shoulder is truly liberating and will change the tone of your conversations! You can also position yourself square to your main workstation while carrying on a conversation or answering calls. Try switching to a laptop computer if you can; its position is easily shifted, you can prop it up on books, change the angle of the screen, even take it with you if you need to lie down.

WEAR SENSIBLE SHOES AND PURSES

Nothing will ruin your back like carrying a heavy load. Don't fool yourself into thinking a purse is not heavy enough to cause problems. Purses are almost always held on one side or the other and the asymmetry causes problems. Think about temporarily trading in your purse for a fanny pack or a stylish mini-backpack. As

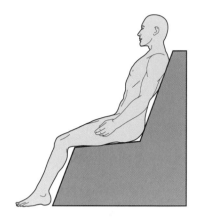

▲ Lean back about 70 degrees to rest your back. Spine pressure is reduced by the transfer of upper body weight to the chair back.

Disc Pressure from Activities[3, 4]

Lying on back	25 kg
Standing	100 kg
Bending forward	150 kg
Slouching in chair	180 kg
A full sit-up	210 kg

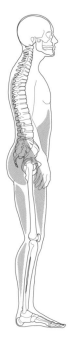

▲ Standing posture, a side view.

What's New: Discs Under Pressure

Although there has been recent controversy in terms of whether sitting disc pressures are actually higher than standing disc pressures, the details are important.[5] Studies have shown that slouching forward when sitting increases disc pressures by an additional 50 percent. Leaning back into the seat back will transfer weight from the upper body to the seat-back and will further reduce disc pressures.

198

a guideline, don't carry a bag that is heavier than you can lift with a single finger. You may need to hold off on toting around your laptop, or trade in for a netbook. Even better, put the battery pack into a rolling bag when travelling.

Wear the best athletic shoes you can afford. Consider buying shoes a size larger and adding in a high-density insole; several are available at your local drug store. These range in price up to $20 but are worth the expense in terms of protecting your back from the repeated micro-trauma of walking all day on hard floors. Never underestimate the importance of good footwear to your overall program of recovery from back pain. Getting into the right shoes with the proper amount of cushioning can make a real difference. If you add inserts to your shoes, make sure your toes and instep still have wiggle room. You can easily identify potential pressure points by wearing a new pair of shoes for 2 hours, then inspecting the foot for red spots. Sometimes minor adjustments can be made at the shoe retailer or cobbler.

DON'T STAND STILL

Remember that standing is not a static activity.[6] In addition to shifting your weight back and forth, front and back, try to sit down for a few minutes. Do some stretches, lunges, and calf stretches if you're waiting for someone or something. A mat in front of the kitchen sink can relieve some of the strain that comes with dish washing and other food prep tasks. If you have no balance problems, the kitchen can be a great place for stretching your leg and hip muscles; the counter edge makes a great balance bar. But if you have a history of falls or are finding balance to be a problem, be mindful that kitchen floors can be unforgiving surfaces to land on.

SQUEEZE THE SHOULDER BLADES TO COUNTERACT THE HUNCH

Holding your arms at your sides, bend your elbows so that your hands level with your elbows. Now pull your elbows back as if you are trying to bring them toward the center of the back. As you do this, your shoulder blades will come towards each other. Go with this and try to tighten these muscles and hold for several seconds. Rest and repeat four more times. The feeling of the shoulder blades moving together occurs with the tightening of two muscles called the rhomboids. Strengthening the rhomboids will help reverse the effects of prolonged sitting, reading, and hunching over paperwork.

WALL SLIDES HELP BUILD LEG STRENGTH FOR LIFTING

You should always ask your doctor and your physical therapist before you resume lifting after an injury. If you must, try to lift objects that are positioned at a waist-high location. Proper lifting involves keeping the spine as vertical as possible and using the muscles of the thighs and buttocks. This means that you won't be ready to lift until your legs are strong enough to support you as you bend down deeply. If you are not used to this kind of bending, it can be very hard on the knees, but as you get stronger, it will become easier. One exercise that is helpful in re-establishing the needed muscles is the wall slide exercise. (See page 103). Always remember that in order to pick up objects safely, you must bend at the knees and keep your bottom low; lift with the legs. Whenever possible get help, and if a lot of lifting is needed, weigh the advantages of hiring someone to do it.

The Explanation

The central purpose of ergonomics is to adapt the environment to allow for optimal functioning of the human body, to improve people's tolerance for sustained activities and to allow them to live largely pain free. The science of the spine is just beginning to explore the underlying mechanisms that explain why it's so important to maintain good body mechanics all the time.[7]

The spine is held together by muscles, tendons, joints, and ligaments. When we slouch over or lean forward, the ligaments that normally bind the bones are placed under strain. Yes, the ligaments will work hard to hold the spine in position, but even 20 minutes of strain on the spinal ligaments will result in lasting over-stretch of the ligament that is measurable over a day later.[8] The significance of the overstretched ligaments is that they lead to back muscle hyper-excitability, muscle spasm, and ultimately, pain.

Get Up for 10 Minutes of Every Hour

At first, it may be overly ambitious to sit for 50 minutes. If you have just had a back injury, you may not be able to sit at all. Sometimes, it's the transition from lying to any other position that is especially painful. If you are in the very acute stages of a back injury, don't push yourself to do much sitting, especially if it is excruciatingly painful. Once you are recovered enough to sit for a period, make sure you learn to recognize how long this period may be. When pain begins to ramp up, stop sitting and note how long you were able to sit comfortably for. You may need to set a timer to make sure you don't overdo it. Once you have made an excellent recovery, you will still need to take breaks every hour to prevent muscle strain and atrophy.

CHAPTER RESOURCES

1. Pope, Malcolm H. 2004. Bernardino Ramazzin. *Spine* 29 (20): 2335-8.

2. Hedge, A. "Ergonomics, Anthropometrics, Biomechanics," http://ergo.human.cornell.edu. Accessed February 10, 2010.

3. Nachemson, A.L. 1976. The lumbar spine: An orthopedic challenge. *Spine* 1:59-71.

4. Finneson, B.E. *Low Back Pain, Second edition*. Philadelphia, PA: JB Lippincott, 1980.

5. Claus, A., et al. 2008. Sitting versus standing. *Journal of Electromyography and Kinesiology* 18: 550-558.

6. Boccia, F.J. *Mindfulness Yoga*. Boston, MA: Wisdom Publications, 2004.

7. Hertling, D. and R.M. Kessler. *Management of Common Musculoskeletal Disorders*. Philadelphia, PA: Lippincott Williams & Wilkins, 2006.

8. Solomonow, M. 2004. Ligaments. *Journal of Electromyography and Kinesiology* 14: 49-60.

CHAPTER 17

Better Nights, Better Days: Sleep and Intimacy

Simple, inexpensive bedding can make sleep and sex significantly more comfortable.

the DIAGNOSIS

> Do you wake up in the morning feeling like you've been run over by a truck?

> Do you wake up in the middle of the night unable to sleep because of back pain?

> Is your bad back ruining your sex life?

Restful sleep is essential for normal alertness and function during the day. Yet pain is increasingly recognized as a major cause of sleep disruption. Whether you are a life-long insomniac, someone who intermittently experiences disrupted sleep, or a relative newcomer to being awake in the wee hours, you will find helpful guidance in this chapter.

And sleep is not the only thing you do in bed. Regardless of how traditional or non-traditional a life-partnership may be, the need to experience the mutual joys of sexual fulfillment are indisputable. Physical intimacy can be a wonderful source of renewal and reassurance. If you have back pain, your sex life is going to face some challenges. The second part of this chapter will explore some ideas in this area.

the **PRESCRIPTION**

FOR BETTER SLEEP:

- Choose a well-constructed mattress or futon topped with two or more layers of foam. Add a soft pillow and leg support pillows to ease back strain.
- If you're currently having back pain, make sure to take some pain medicine one to two hours before bed so that you are as comfortable as possible at bedtime.
- Engage in soothing activities before bedtime. Avoid caffeine or vigorous exercise in the evening.
- Minimize non-sleep activities in the bedroom. If you can't sleep, get up and do something quietly in another room.
- As much as possible, restrict sleeping to the nighttime hours.

FOR A BETTER LOVE LIFE:

- You will need to gently let your partner know what works best and what you are afraid might hurt. You may have to try out some new positions or alternative ways of sharing physical pleasure in order to avoid making back pain worse. Most authorities recommend that the person with back pain avoid the top position.[1]
- Use reliable strategies for pain mitigation before and after sex. Try taking a warm bath or cozying up with the heating pad ahead of time. Afterwards, you may need to treat your back with an ice pack. So as not to spoil the fleeting pleasures of the after-glow, you can have this wrapped in a towel and handy at the bedside even before beginning.

The Treatment

Proper sleep allows the body and mind to recharge. You spend nearly a third of your life sleeping, so it makes sense to invest some time, energy, and resources into improving your sleep experience. Are you sleeping on a mattress that was top-of-the-line when you bought it 20 years ago? Has it been more than six months since you turned and rotated your mattress? Are you waking up in the middle of the night with aching joints? Are you falling asleep during the day and lying awake at night? Answering yes to these questions indicates the need to take a hard look at your sleeping arrangements. Experienced people with back trouble know the benefits of a proper sleep environment.

START WITH A FIRM MATTRESS

Your choice of mattress has a big impact on your ability to sleep well when living with back pain. You want a mattress that is firm enough to provide good support for the heaviest parts of your body, but one that offers some resilience to accommodate the body's natural curves.[2] A spring coil mattress is a good start, but many people prefer the feel of a futon. Either way, you will need to add some cushioning at least initially during the back recovery process. When you are recovering from a back injury, it may be necessary to lie still for longer than you were previously used to—first, because it may be painful to change position too often; second, because it may be necessary to rest your spine by holding a particular position; and third, because sleep positions that you used to enjoy may not be comfortable.

PAD YOUR NEST FOR MORE REST

The need for padding on top of a firm mattress cannot be underestimated. The number of patients who initially express skepticism about this simple change is pretty large, and the number who deliver enthusiastic feedback is nearly as large. In fact, if you can do one thing to make your life with back pain better, it is to invest a few dollars in cushioning your firm mattress. The key here is to go for more rather than less; not more money—more layers.

The best thing to do is to buy a king-sized egg-crate style foam pad and fold it over a few times until it is the size of your sleeping area on your bed. You may wind up with two, three, or four layers of foam. The most common mistake that people make is to add only a single layer. This is not enough. Start by adding four layers of foam and cut back if it feels too cushy. A high-quality mattress cover will reduce the sense of limited breathability that people sometimes experience when lying on foam mattress pads.

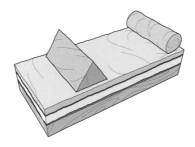

▲ A better bed. Use a wedge pillow or other support for your legs.

What's New: Futons Cause More Pain

Recent research has shown that sleeping on a hard mattress, such as a futon, is associated with more pain in people with low back pain. If you own a futon, add an egg-crate style mattress pad, folded to create at least two layers over the futon.

The second mistake that people make is to get too fancy. By this, I mean investing hundreds of dollars in the latest high-tech foam product available. Generally speaking, a couple of egg-crate style foam pads are better than the super-expensive high-tech foam pads and are a lot less expensive! The egg-crate style foam pads will not last, though; after a few months, you will want to rotate the pieces from high pressure zones of the body (under the hips) to other areas and extend the life of a foam pad for another year.

A soft, supportive pillow for the head and neck will make it easier to lie on your back during the night and can be folded over if needed for side-lying. Again, a modest investment will make a big difference in your nighttime and daytime comfort levels. Test some different pillows and shop for sales so that you can go with the top-of-the-line if needed. If you don't like a particular pillow for your head, you can always rotate it to support your legs or arms.

While recovering from back pain, you will need to use a support pillow or wedge for the legs. The purpose of this support is to put the spine into a position of rest. Remember that during the day, this involves lying on the back with the legs propped up on a chair or sofa. Most people can achieve this extreme positioning while in bed but some leg support will be helpful. Experiment with different arrangements to determine what works best for you. Some people like just a small roll under the knees, others like a triangular cushion under the knees, and yet others like to have the entire lower leg elevated. One thing to keep in mind is the potential for pressure points. If you are propping up the knees, it might increase pressure on the heels or on the buttock. This doesn't mean you should give up on a leg-supported sleeping arrangement; it just means that further adjustment is necessary. Your goal is to find a sleeping arrangement that feels comfortable and healthful.

YOUR SLEEP ENVIRONMENT: PUTTING THE PIECES TOGETHER

Most people enjoy sleeping in clean, soft sheets. If your back pain is more severe at the moment, you may need help changing the sheets and getting the laundry done. It's always okay to ask for help, but it's even more okay if you're sure to ask graciously and express appreciation. Most people like to help but most also like to know that their help is noted.

You will want to create a bedroom space that is conducive to sleep. Ideally, there should not be a television or computer in the bedroom. Exercise equipment should be set up somewhere else. Make sure that there is no excess light entering the room during your sleeping hours; you may need to purchase a light-blocking shade or some room-darkening curtains. To the extent possible, insist on quiet during sleep times. You may need to purchase some earplugs; even inexpensive earplugs are very effective and can really help ensure deeper, more restful sleep.

Go to bed only when you're sleepy. This may mean staying up a little bit past bedtime, but it's better to hit the pillow ready to sleep than to lie down with the problems of the world swirling around in your mind. Sometimes it's helpful to develop a pre-bedtime routine. A warm bath, a hot cup of tea, a favorite book of calculus—well, maybe not calculus—can all help bring on feelings of calm and comfort. There are evening yoga routines and meditation practices that help ready the mind for sleep. An evening session of Qi Gong can help clear the thoughts and bring on a sense of serenity before bedtime.

Always make yourself get up on time. If you're having trouble sleeping at night, snoozing late into the morning will only push the problem forward to the next night. If you are troubled by insomnia, resist the temptation to sleep in on weekends and stringently avoid daytime naps. Nothing will wreck nighttime sleep like an afternoon siesta. If you are not troubled by nighttime wakefulness, nap away—but there is a growing sense that proper sleep patterns are necessary for overall health and longevity.

Make conscious choices during the day to improve your sleep at night. This includes getting some moderately vigorous exercise each day but avoiding such exercise in the four-to-five hours before bedtime. Cut back on caffeine or eliminate it altogether. Studies have shown that cutting out caffeine not only makes it easier to fall asleep, but lengthens sleep duration and improves sleep quality.[3] Drink alcohol only in moderation and avoid it altogether while taking medication for back pain. Although coffee liqueurs are popular with younger drinkers, they have disastrous effects on sleep initiation and maintenance.

Intimacy with Back Pain

Keeping in touch with your intimate partner during an experience of back pain is also important to getting better quickly. Modern strategies for coping with persistent pain recognize the importance of incorporating pleasurable activities into everyday life.[4] Sex is an important part of how adults play and find enjoyment. It's important to do what you can to keep this a positive force in your life.

However, acute pain can interfere with a person's sex drive. So if you're in the midst of a severe bout of back pain, don't expect miracles. If you are receiving treatment with prescription medications for chronic back pain, be aware that many of these medications can interfere with libido and performance. This may be a good reason to pursue the non-pharmacological approaches to treating back pain more aggressively.

Float on a Warm Water Bed

If you love the feel of a water bed, this is another alternative for people with back pain. However if you're not used to this kind of mattress, it can be difficult and intimidating to get into and out of. Water mattresses are often temperature controlled, making it possible to benefit from some thermal therapy while sleeping.

205

PACE YOURSELF

The first part of pacing for better sex is to know when to jump back into the game. If it's too soon to return to heavy action, your body will let you know. One way to get better results is to slow down and enjoy each moment as it happens. Watch a movie together; sit a little closer than usual, try massaging your partner's shoulders or feet. All of these things can bring you together and let you acknowledge the importance of staying physically connected while making adjustments for back pain. Part of pacing is making sure that you're allocating enough time for sex to happen at an easy pace. This can be difficult with work, school, family, and friends all competing for your time. Don't let your love life be the victim.

Anticipation is where much of the most intense pleasure in life is found. Think back to your childhood years. The incredible yearning that preceded your favorite holiday or a special birthday, the happy anticipation of knowing that summer vacation was coming at last. Especially when trying to adjust to back pain or to live through an episode of back pain, building on the anticipation of sex is a pain-free way to extend the enjoyment of your experience. Of course, anticipation is really only fun for most people if there is a genuine reward in the end, so it's important not to overextend the anticipation phase and end up with empty exasperation. Anticipation and fulfillment are both important for most people.

MEANINGFUL WORDS AND ACTIONS

We all have special signals or triggers that speak most clearly to us. Some people love a good strong hug, others deeply relish a cup of coffee in the morning, a home-cooked meal, or tickets to the new show in town. In life, it's critically important to know not only your own deepest desires are but also to understand the inner heart of your intimate partner. Is this someone who comes home exhausted and would love 15 minutes to lie down before starting the evening together, or is this a person who gets home ready to run full tilt? Is this someone who gets a thrill from seeing a new outfit, or is the old and familiar better and more attractive? Are whispered sentiments of affection cloying or the start of an exciting night together? The key to increasing happiness in a relationship is understanding what your partner most deeply values and bringing that forward to the extent that you can. Make every moment really count by speaking to your partner in words and actions that are most meaningful. You will add life to your years.

AMP IT UP WITH FANTASY OR SCENTS

Adding an element of fantasy to your intimate relationship is a great way to have fun as adults. You can do this simply and with a light-hearted touch. The ideal is not to have the other person fulfill your fantasy but rather to spark a new series of imaginations that arise spontaneously for both of you. What works best will depend on you and your partner. Some people are more responsive to music, others to food, and still others to clothing. It is often said that variety is the spice of life, but playful variations of the familiar are where greater enjoyment is found for most people.

Pleasing scents can play an important role in creating mood and setting the pace for an intimate encounter. The fragrances that stimulate male and female responses are not always the same. Lavender has been shown to create a state of relaxation and arousal for women. Men may respond more strongly to the scents of vanilla and orange as positive signals. You can incorporate scents in your love life in many different ways: perfumed massage oils, scented candles, sachets tucked into a pillow case, as a soothing bath beforehand, or the recently popularized room fragrance sprays. A little dab of essential oil onto various parts of the body can have a powerful positive effect. Music can either sooth or inspire the object of your desire; consider creating a bit of ambience with your loved one's favorite tunes.

SAFE POSITIONS FOR ACHING BACKS

The actual doing of sexual intercourse may require some adjustments during an episode of back pain.[5] The ordinary activities of intercourse can involve movements of the spine and pelvis that are frankly pain-provoking and may make things worse rather than better. It is generally held that the person with back pain should take the lower position. If you can arrange things so that the spine is supported as you lie on your back, this is usually ideal. A pillow underneath the buttocks can be supportive while further improving the mechanics a bit.[6] A good alternative for many people is to start with the person who has back pain taking up a side-lying position. This can accommodate a variety of relative positions from the partner. Women who are experiencing back pain will often find that a posterior entry position is more problematic because of the extension or arching of the spine that this entails. When returning to intercourse after an episode of particularly severe back pain, begin slowly at first and limit encounters to relatively shorter sessions until experience shows just how much activity is tolerable without provoking pain. Consider researching this area a bit, as there are several recommended books on the market.

PREPARATION AND RECOVERY

You may want to prepare ahead of time with a hot shower, warm bath, or a 20-minute session with the heating pad. This will have the effect of increasing relaxation, loosening up the necessary muscles, and decreasing pain. Afterwards, it is usually a good idea to treat your back to some ice. Sex is oftentimes just like having a good workout, in terms of the physical demands that are placed on the back and spine. Treat it like you would any other physical exertion. An icepack wrapped in cloth applied to the back will make your memories happy ones and decrease your chance of persisting pain afterwards.

The Explanation

It's a catch-22: pain will disrupt sleep, and disrupted sleep will amplify pain. More and more studies are showing that getting pain under control is very important to reduce sleep disruption in a lot of people with ongoing musculoskeletal problems such as arthritis. Disrupted sleep also interferes with a person's capacity to cope with pain and make good decisions about how to best manage an ongoing pain problem.

Most people do not get sufficient sleep. The normal amount of sleep needed is eight hours. Most of us are running around getting substantially less. This is because we budget eight hours into our busy schedule for sleep, which makes the false assumption that sleep begins immediately upon lying down and ends at the prescribed moment in the morning. To the extent possible, you should allow more time for sleep rather than less. Especially when recovering from a back problem, your body needs time to heal. The more chances you can give yourself to get a good night's rest, the better you will be overall.

CHAPTER RESOURCES

1. White, A.A. and A.E. White. *Back Care, 2nd Edition*. Issaquah, WA: Medic Publishing Co., 1996.

2. Bergholdt, K., et al. 2008. Better backs by better beds? *Spine* 33 (7): 703-708.

3. Sin, C.W., J.S. Ho, and J.W. Chung. 2009. Systematic review on the effectiveness of caffeine abstinence on the quality of sleep. *J Clin Nurs* 18 (1): 13-21.

4. Otis, J.D. *Managing Chronic Pain, A Cognitive-Behavioral Therapy Approach*. New York: Oxford University Press, 2007.

5. Maigne, J.Y. and G. Chatellier. 2001. Assessment of sexual activity in patients with back pain compared with patients with neck pain. *Clin Orthop Relat Res* 385:82-7.

6. White, A.A. and A.E. White. *Back Care, 2nd Edition*. Issaquah, WA: Medic Publishing Co., 1996.

If I can't sleep because of my back pain, should I take a sleeping pill?

Many people have turned to medications to improve sleep. You will notice that none of the recommendations in this chapter include anything about drugs for sleep. As a rule, drugs for sleep are a temporary solution. They are also, by and large, a bandage over a problem that really needs more serious fixing. If you must ask your doctor for sleep medicines, do so, but recognize that taking a pill before addressing the fundamentals of good sleep hygiene is a fool's wager. Ask yourself about the quality of your sleep; see if you really feel better the next morning after taking a sleeping pill. If not, start making better choices that allow for natural sleep to occur.

CHAPTER 18

Massage and Acupuncture for Back Pain

Highly effective therapies without the side effects of medication.

the DIAGNOSIS

> Do you have chronic muscle tension in your back?

> Are you walking around feeling like you're just not yourself anymore?

If you answered yes to these two questions, there are two things you should do right away: 1) undertake a trial of massage and/or acupuncture and 2) fix your daily ergonomics (Chapter 16).

Massage and acupuncture usually don't get the credit they deserve as potentially effective therapies without the side effects of most medications. Massage especially is generally safe and will result in almost immediate pain relief. Acupuncture is also widely practiced and usually requires significant training on the part of the practitioner. Still, in some places, people can become licensed in acupuncture with only 200 hours of training (five weeks full time), but obviously it takes a lot longer to become truly skillful at this technique. To pursue acupuncture, you will want to start with a recommendation from someone local who's had good experience with this treatment.

How Long Will the Benefits Last?

You may have heard from naysayers that massage only helps for a little while, and the next day the pain will be back. This might be true in some cases, but for certain problems—such as sudden muscle injury from a car accident or a sporting mishap—massage can fix the problem in one or a few sessions. Some conditions such as spinal degeneration or muscle spasm compounded by nerve compression may take longer to accrue lasting benefits.

Ask your massage therapist or acupuncturist if they have any recommendations to ensure the maximum benefit from therapy. Many times it's prudent to take a short nap and go easy for the rest of the day, but sometimes this isn't practical. If your massage or acupuncture treatments don't seem to be working the way you think they should, make sure you're following through after each session and not just jumping back into your life at breakneck speed.

More and more people are looking to alternative therapies as a way to circumvent the potential problems that come with medication and surgery. Among the most effective treatments are trigger point massage and acupuncture. Other therapies such as cranial-sacral massage and myofascial release are very popular in some locales.

- If you haven't tried back massage for your back pain, make an appointment with a qualified massage therapist in your area and give it a try.
- Check out a book on trigger point techniques. The best available is Clair Davies's *Trigger Point Therapy Workbook*. Other books include Simeon Niel-Asher's beautifully illustrated paperback guide and Travell and Simons's encyclopedic work, but few match Davies for clarity and inclusiveness.[1,2,3]
- Call your insurance company to determine if it will provide coverage for massage or acupuncture. Insurance coverage for alternative therapies varies widely. Some larger companies include acupuncture in their range of benefits; some states even require this coverage. Check to make sure that a failure to meet pre-conditions for coverage, such as obtaining a doctor's prescription, won't prevent you from getting the claim paid.
- Ask your friends and family if they know someone who performs acupuncture and what their experience was like. Although the thought of having acupuncture needles inserted can be a bit intimidating, the needles are always sterile and precision manufactured to produce as little pain as possible. Most of the time, there is very little pain associated with the acupuncture treatment itself. Sometimes a mild burning sensation is all that is felt.
- Consider trying acupressure. Acupressure uses self-massage techniques to stimulate the flow of Qi (energy in the body) by pressing particular points on the body. One method of acupressure for relief of back pain is described in this chapter, but you may want to consult a specialist to learn more.

The Treatment

There are many options for massage therapy, including trigger point massage, myofascial release, cranio-sacral work, and acupressure. Acupuncture is an ancient Eastern therapy that continues to make inroads in the West. Massage is especially helpful in the first few weeks of a pain problem, as it can interrupt the vicious cycle of pain leading to spasm leading to more pain. Once the muscles are relaxed via massage, normal blood flow can return and healing can resume.

TRIGGER POINT MASSAGE RELEASES TENSION

If your doctor recommends a trial of massage for your back pain, seek out someone skilled in trigger point methods. You may find that your physical therapist is already using these approaches on your back. Trigger point massage is an offshoot of one of the most effective approaches to addressing musculoskeletal pain: trigger point therapy.

You can take one of two approaches to trigger point massage: let someone else do it or do it yourself. Trigger point therapy for the back is a bit tricky for the newcomer, although there are products such as the "theracane" that are designed to make it easy to get to inaccessible points on the back, lower leg, and shoulders. One low-tech approach that works well is to put one or two racquetball balls into a sock and dangle the sock behind you as you move back and forth against a wall.[4] These D-I-Y approaches will probably work better once you've had a chance to learn about trigger points and become familiar with the basic process through the experience of receiving professional trigger point therapy. Although practitioners will use a variety of techniques to release trigger points, including the use of acupuncture needles, injection of local anesthetics, and spraying with a freezy-cold aerosol, you can actually learn to apply pressure to the muscle and train yourself to relax the muscles on cue. The pressure itself, when correctly applied, will induce a relaxation response in the muscle trigger point.

Trigger points were described by Dr. Janet Travell as having four essential features: 1) a palpable tight band within the muscle, 2) a focused spot of tenderness within the tight band, 3) reproduction of pain in a nearby part of the body when the tight band is compressed by pressure from the fingers, and 4) relaxation of the tight band with proper massage technique.[5] Once someone is trained to feel trigger points, it becomes immediately apparent that many people are walking around with trigger points, some of which produce pain and others that don't seem to be bothersome at all. The non-bothersome trigger points are referred to as *latent*, and the trigger points that produce pain are called *active*.[6]

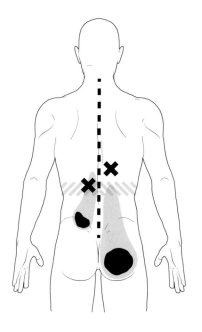

▲ Referred pain. Trigger point massage helps relieve tension in your back.

213

What's New: Recognition of Pulsating Spinal Fluid

There has been little support for cranio-sacral therapy published in the standard medical literature.[7] However, most medical practitioners have been slow to recognize that there is a patterned flow of spinal fluid through the central spinal canal. Further, the fact that the flow of spinal fluid is pulsatile has only recently been more widely acknowledged.

One feature of trigger points is that they are not only painful directly when pressed upon, but they also result in pain at a distance. This is probably because of the way muscles travel from one part to another, as the hamstring muscles travel from hip to knee, but may also have to do with other features of the body's pain sensing system. This sets trigger points apart from an ordinary muscle spasm. For example, a trigger point in the calf can produce ankle or foot pain. This may be because that calf muscle has a tendon that extends into the foot but could have to do with nerve compressions or other problems. As you learn about your back, you will come to know that many of the muscles in the back are associated with pain that's actually in the muscle. One back muscle, the quadratus lumborum, connects the top of the hip bone to the ribcage. Its trigger point pain syndrome results in sacroiliac pain.

MYOFASCIAL RELEASE LOOSENS FIBROUS CONNECTIONS

Myofascial release massage is based on the idea that fibrous connections build up between adjacent tissues that are not subjected to full and vigorous movements. Over time, these fibrous connections progressively tighten and shorten. This process leads to worsening stiffness and restrictions in movement that can lead to abnormal movement patterns becoming entrenched and leading to chronic pain.[8] The overall objective of myofascial release massage is to release these fibrous connections, leading to freer, fuller, and less painful movements. This is accomplished through a serious of kneading, rolling, and deep pressure movements. Myofascial release massage can feel a bit strange as it focuses on the "spaces between the muscles" rather than working on the muscles themselves at some phases of the massage. It may be combined with other forms of massage, but can have tremendously beneficial effects in and of itself.

The word *myofascial* is derived from a combination of *myo*, meaning muscle, and *fascial*, meaning fascia. Fascia is a fibrous connective tissue in the body. Fine and weblike in some places, fascia can also be very strong and tough in some parts of the body. Fascia has been described as being like plastic wrap, in that it is normally nice and smooth.[9] When one section of the fascia is entrapped by abnormal fibrous attachments to a body part (muscle, internal organ, etc.), this produces a distortion in the fascia that tugs or pulls on another body part and will restrain normal movements. Pain is the inevitable result. Myofascial release uses a series of pulling or stretching movements to loosen these abnormal fibrous bands. As usually practiced, it requires the therapist to listen carefully to what his or her hands perceive and to adjust the treatment to address each person's trouble spots.

Rolfing is a structured approach to myofascial release that leads to a state of structural integration.[10] The goal of rolfing is to correct abnormalities in musculo-skeletal alignment and reorient the various body segments so they are aligned with the earth's gravitational field. Once upon a time, rolfing was conducted in a very vigorous manner and the resulting therapy experience was sometimes painful, although with good results. More recently, rolfing practitioners have focused on accomplishing the goals of myofascial release and structural re-alignment in a more tolerable manner. In general, rolfing follows a specific sequence of techniques to systematically release myofascial adhesions, beginning with the feet and working upwards through various body parts.

CRANIO-SACRAL MASSAGE MANIPULATES THE SKELETON

Cranio-sacral therapy arose at the turn of the twentieth century out of a postulate about the relative motion of skull and sacrum, and ideas about the flow of spinal fluid through the brain and spinal cord. The idea that the bones of the adult skull can move and are subject to manipulation is inconsistent with published research. Yet cranio-sacral therapy appears to be safe. It is performed using light touch while a person is resting, fully clothed, on the back. Through gentle application of pressure and re-positioning of the head, shoulders, spine, pelvis, hips, and back, the cranio-sacral therapist seeks to re-establish subtle rhythms of the body.

ACUPRESSURE MASSAGE INCREASES THE BODY'S ENERGY

Acupressure massage utilizes the philosophy of energy (Qi) from Chinese medicine to map out a series of pressure points on the body that, when compressed properly, are believed to stimulate the flow of Qi. Originating more than 5,000 years ago, acupressure actually was practiced before acupuncture, which required the development of needles, and more recently, electrical stimulation methodologies.[11] The location of acupressure points is established based on a series of meridians that map out the flow of Qi through the body.[12]

Acupressure is widely used for the treatment of back pain. Several approaches can be used. One popular technique for back pain involves placing pressure on a on a spot located on either side of the spine at about the waist level. This point is sometimes identified as the B23 spot.[13] You can locate the spot as follows: Sit upright on the edge of a chair or stand with feet shoulder width apart. Hold out your hands, palm side downwards with the thumb sticking out from the hand. Now position your hands so that they are touching your waist on either side, your thumb should be lightly touching your back and your elbows sticking out to the

Warning! Jelly May Roll

Make sure to check with your massage therapist about recommendations for activity after myofascial release massage. Following a vigorous session, you may be a little more loosely held together than usual. Vigorous or especially effortful activities may result in inadvertent muscle strains as your movement patterns will shift immediately after this treatment.

The Miracle Ball

The miracle ball is a product designed to apply just the right amount of pressure to the body. The idea behind the miracle ball is that in order for pressure to work, it has to have not only the right firmness, but also the right geometry. The miracle ball attempts to solve both of these challenges. Usually provided as a pair, they are about four inches (10 cm) in diameter and made of resilient plastic. When properly inflated, the miracle balls are fairly firm and can support the weight of the body as you lay on them. The balls come with a guide book, which is very helpful in terms of describing the different ways in which the balls can be used for relief of neck and back pain. Mid-back and sacroiliac pain may also respond to treatment with the miracle balls.

side. Move your hands closer to the midline of your back, still holding them in the palm-down position, until your thumbs are about three inches apart from each other on either side of the spine. You've been applying very light pressure to the skin with the thumbs until now. At this point you will increase the pressure that the thumbs are applying by pressing your elbows backward and arching the back gently. In applying this pressure, you should not feel pain of any significance. You may feel that the muscles underlying the skin are firm or soft; the pressure may be completely painless or feel as though there is some tension. Hold this pressure for several seconds, or two to three minutes if it seems helpful. A similar technique is described in Lee Holden's book *7 Minutes of Magic: The Ultimate Energy Workout*.[14] If your back pain worsens with this procedure, stop immediately. This description should not be read as a recommendation of medical therapy in any sense, and is provided here only to open up new possibilities in your self-management of back pain. You should always have your back pain fully evaluated for serious causes by a qualified health professional.

SWEDISH MASSAGE USES RELAXING STROKES

Swedish massage (sometimes called classical massage) is a traditional massage modality that uses specific massage strokes to produce an overall sense of relaxation and well-being. There are five types of massage strokes used in Swedish massage, ranging from fingertip pressure to deep, kneading pressure. Everyone is a little different, and you may find that Swedish massage is right for you.

ACUPUNCTURE SHIFTS THE BODY'S ENERGY FLOW

Acupuncture has generally gained acceptance as a potentially helpful treatment for a variety of disorders, chief among which is back pain. Surveys have shown that more than three million Americans have used acupuncture in the last year and that this is increasing.[15] It could be the topic of a very long book (or several books), but a few words here will have to suffice.

Acupuncture is based on the Eastern belief system of shifting energy flows in the body. The energy flows are organized into meridians that run through the limbs and torso and are mainly named for various internal organs: lung, large intestine, stomach, spleen, heart, small intestine, bladder, kidney, pericardium, gallbladder, liver, and triple warmer.[16] These twelve meridians and an additional two channels (the conception vessel and the governor vessel) make 14 in total.

In modern practice, very thin, sterile needles that are precision manufactured are inserted into the body through the skin. The sensation of acupuncture varies with the treatment plan and the insertion site; however, the actual placement of needles can be painless. The number of needles used will vary but one aspect that strikes Westerners as unusual is the emphasis on placing needles in delicate structures such as the outer ear and the nose. Although acupuncture can be performed while the patient is seated when appropriate, most of the time acupuncture is carried out while someone is lying down.

The Explanation

Although the use of massage for the treatment of back pain is often dismissed as unproven, ineffective, or soft science, massage plays an important role for many people with back injury or back pain.[17] Its value depends on at least three factors: the nature of the back problem itself, the personality and inclinations of the person with the back problem, and the type of massage that is being used for treatment. For massage to be successful, all three factors have to be aligned with each other and the skill of the massage therapist as well.

As a first point, most back problems will not be worsened by massage, but the exceptions to this rule are quite serious and when unrecognized could lead to consequences as serious as spinal cord injury and permanent nerve damage. Conditions such as fracture of the vertebra or spinal abscess should not be treated by massage, as this could either worsen the damage or needlessly delay essential treatment. These caveats aside, the management of most back injury problems will be complemented and even greatly enhanced by massage. The reason for this is simple: even back problems which are not primarily muscular to begin with often evolve to have a component of muscle spasms as a significant source of pain and disability.

What's New: Belief in Acupuncture Matters

The scientific evidence in support of acupuncture is patchy. There are studies that claim to show a benefit for specific conditions, such as dental pain and arthritis of the knee, and then there are other studies that show no benefit at all. One recent study of back pain showed that acupuncture was better than placebo, but it also showed that simulated acupuncture was helpful and not any worse than the real thing.[18] Several studies have indicated that the patient's expectations for acupuncture have a major impact on the outcome.[19] Put into plain language, if you think it will work, it probably will. For some it might seem like an expensive sugar pill, but for those who believe in acupuncture, the pain relieving effects are phenomenal.

CHAPTER RESOURCES

1. Simons, D.G., J.G. Travell, and L.S. Simons. *Travell and Simons' Myofascial Pain and Dysfunction: The Trigger Point Manual. 2nd Edition.* Baltimore, MD: Williams & Wilkins, 1999.

2. Niel-Asher, S. *The Concise Book of Trigger Points, Revised Edition.* Berkeley, CA: North Atlantic Books, 2008.

3. Davies, C. *The Trigger Point Therapy Workbook.* Oakland (CA): New Harbinger Publications, Inc., 2001.

4. Ibid.

5. Wilson, V.P. 2003. Janet G. Travell, MD: A daughter's recollection. *Tex Heart Inst J* 30 (1): 8-12.

Warning! New Needles Required

Acupuncture is generally very safe, and the major risks of infection or perforation of a major organ are rare.[20] Because re-using acupuncture needles could result in the transmission of serious illnesses, it is important to receive acupuncture from a reputable practitioner and to be certain that the needles used on you are coming from a freshly opened (sterile) package.

6. Shah, J.P., et al. 2008. Biochemicals associated with pain and inflammation are elevated in sites near to and remote from active myofascial trigger points. *Arch Phys Med Rehabil* 89 (1): 16-23.

7. Downey, P.A., T. Barbano, R. Kapur-Wadhwa, J.J. Sciote, M.I. Siegel, and M.P. Mooney. 2006. Craniosacral therapy: The effects of cranial manipulation on intracranial pressure and cranial bone movement. *J Orthop Sports Phys Ther* 36 (11): 845-53.

8. Finley, J.E. "Myofascial Pain," eMedicine. http://emedicine.medscape.com/article/313007-overview. Accessed January, 24 2010.

9. Manheim, C.J. *The Myofascial Release Manual.* Thorofare, New Jersey: SLACK Inc., 2008.

10. Rolf, I.P. *Rolfing: Reestablishing the Natural Alignment and Structural Integration of the Human Body for Vitality and Well-Being.* Rochester: Healing Arts Press, 1989.

11. Gach, M. *Acupressure's Potent Points.* New York: Bantam Books, 1990.

12. NIH. "Acupuncture for Pain," http://nccam.nih.gov/health/acupuncture/acupuncture-for-pain.htm. Accessed January, 24 2010.

13. Averoff, S.E. Acupressure and Reflex Points for Common Ailments, http://www.lind.com/quantum/acupoints%20for%20good%20health.htm. Accessed January, 24 2010.

14. Holden, L. *7 Minutes of Magic.* New York: Penguin Group (USA) Inc., 2007.

15. Burke, A., D.M. Upchurch, C. Dye, and L. Chyu. 2006. Acupuncture use in the United States: Findings from the National Health Interview Survey. *J Altern Complement Med* 12 (7): 639-48.

16. Hecker, H.-U., A. Steveling, E. Peuker, J. Kastner, and K. Liebchen. *Color Atlas of Acupuncture.* New York: Thieme, 2001.

17. Furlan, A.D., M. Imamura, T. Dryden, and E. Irvin. 2009. Massage for low back pain: An updated systematic review within the framework of the Cochrane Back Review Group. *Spine (Phila. Pa, 1976)* 34 (16): 1669-84.

18. Cherkin, et al. 2009. A randomized trial comparing acupuncture, simulated acupuncture, and usual care for chronic low back pain. *Arch Intern Med* 169 (9): 858-66.

19. Kong, J., et al. 2009. An MRI study on the interaction and dissociation between expectation of pain relief and acupuncture treatment. *Neuroimage* 47 (3): 1066-76.

20. Wasan, A.D., et al. 2010. The Impact of Placebo, Psychopathology, and Expectations on the Response to Acupuncture Needling in Patients With Chronic Low Back Pain. *J Pain* [Epub].

Should I use massage oil?

There are many different commercially available oils, creams, and lotions that can be used for massage. In most cases, you will want to perform massage with something to ease the passage of the fingers and hands over the skin. The first criterion for choosing a lubricant is that it not be irritating. Everyone's skin is slightly different, and you may need some trial and error to determine what works best. If you see redness or rash or experience burning after using a certain product, discontinue its use right away. Mineral oil is a petroleum-derived product that is part of many commercially available creams, lotions, and oils. If you want to use something plant-based instead, sweet almond oil is a popular choice that is often available in health food stores.

The second criterion for choosing a massage product is good aesthetics. It is important to note how the product smells and how it feels on the skin. Nowhere is the saying "one man's trash is another man's treasure" more true than when it comes to scents and fragrances. Popular choices include floral scents such as rose, jasmine, or lavender. Herbal scents such as rosemary, menthol, and eucalyptus can give a refreshing feel, and food-based aromas such as vanilla, nutmeg, and orange are soothing to some people.

The material should feel smooth and soothing on the skin. Some people prefer a product the feels invisible, in that very little perceptible awareness of the cream or lotion is felt. There are many products that would like to assert a potential health benefit, but in most cases these claims are tightly regulated. Aside from over-the-counter medicinal creams (such as those containing aspirin-related medications and possibly menthol) typically used for sports injuries, there is little solid evidence to support the use of specific additives to massage products. That said, menthol does have a proven capacity to interfere with pain signals and may be very helpful for some people in relieving their pain. Oregano is very popular with some massage therapists, but oregano oil can be damaging when undiluted and care is needed. Lavender oil has been shown to contain many active compounds, some of which are noted to promote a state of relaxation and pain-relief, and others that have anti-inflammatory effects. Eucalyptus oil may also have active pain-relieving properties, but further studies are needed.

CHAPTER 19

Meditation and Mind/Body Therapies for Pain Control

Focus the mind to relieve back pain and move towards physical wellness.

> **Do you sometimes feel that back pain is ruining your ability to enjoy life?**

> **Do you sometimes feel that life is spiraling out of control since you developed back pain?**

Meditation and other mind-body therapies are one way people can take charge of their own health and wellness. Ultimately, the healthcare choices that we make are an expression of our deeply held values. Unfortunately, many people have the experience that the regular healthcare system is too strongly focused on illness as a state of being, and is designed to generate revenues and not to promote health. This state of affairs is demonstrated by the willingness of insurers to pay $20,000 or more for surgery, but not one cent for massage, meditation, or other alternative therapies. But don't let this be the final arbiter of right and wrong. The choice is yours; you have this book in your hands, and this chapter is written to open your awareness to a healthy new life beyond back pain. If you want to make peace with your back, read on!

Listen to Your Body

Maybe you've had the feeling that your back is a little better when you're on vacation, but you haven't wanted to tell anyone in case they would think your pain is all in your head. It doesn't mean that at all—it just means your body is trying to tell you something about your life, and the message is: It's too much, slow down!

the PRESCRIPTION

One of the best ways to supercharge your recovery from back pain is to pursue health-directed therapies that will reorient your mind's eye toward physical wellness and connect you to people exuding energy, vitality, and enthusiasm. Especially if other therapies have failed to fix the problem, it's time to start thinking outside the box.

- Learn more about meditation and mind-body medicine. Begin with a trip to your public library to find books on the therapies described in this chapter. You can also find information online. The NIH has created a series of fact sheets on alternative therapies.
- Begin to meditate or reinvigorate your practice.
- Talk to your doctor, other healthcare providers, friends, and family about mind-body therapies. Their openness may surprise you.
- Seek out a movement therapy specialist and take a few lessons in Alexander Technique, Feldenkrais, or Qi Gong.
- Consider trying an energy-based therapy such Reiki, which manipulates a person's energy as they remain passive.
- Ask yourself: Is self-hypnosis is worth a try?

The Treatment

Most of the therapies described in this chapter are safe, although for some, question marks remain as to their effectiveness. I will try to point out the limitations of each. In reality though, as many of these therapies require a rather profound level of personal commitment, persistence, and openness to new experience, it will be very difficult to carry out studies that definitively prove a benefit. But again, the choice is yours. For many people, a life centered on mind-body awareness and therapies is a path to peace, happiness, and true productivity.[1]

Meditation Has Proven Benefits

If meditation were a drug, your doctor would be recommending it, your insurance company would be paying for it, and millions of people would be taking it.[2,3] But meditation is not a drug; it is a technique you can master only with determination and effort. There are many approaches to meditation. The key is to start now and remain open-minded about the benefits until you have tried more than one kind of meditation. Although most practitioners and resources advocate meditating one or more times a day, it is possible to obtain benefits from more sporadic meditation.

The basic principle of meditation is to focus the mind to the exclusion of intrusive thoughts.[4] This can either be done through directing all attention to a particular thought (concentration) or by intentionally directing all attention away from particular thoughts (mindfulness). The efficacy of meditation in clinical trials varies, but several studies have reported the benefits of meditative training for back pain. In one study, eight weeks of meditation-based therapy was nearly equivalent to eight weeks of physical therapy in reducing pain and improving quality of life.

The space you chose for meditation is important. It should be as quiet as possible, although some natural background noise is okay. Calm breezes and distant sounds are usually not problematic. If you don't have a space like this, you may want to find some way to create it. There are meditation audio recordings; some people like the sound of a small fountain or a sound-making machine; and noise cancellation headphones might be helpful if outside distractions can't be avoided. The temperature should be comfortable—you will find it hard to meditate effectively if you are chilly, and a cold environment may cause your back muscles to stiffen. Although some religious forms of meditation encourage the use of incense, until your practice develops in a particular direction, it is best to avoid excessive odors, as well as other extremes of sensory input.

What You Need to Meditate

- Quiet space
- 20-45 minutes
- Comfortable position
- A state of wakefulness
- A preferred method

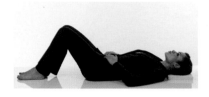

▲ Recumbent meditation position

WHEN ALL ELSE FAILS, MEDITATE

Although the primary purpose of meditation is not to bring order into an over-packed schedule, many people have found that meditation is a way to gently yet firmly reassert control over one's life, experiences, thoughts, and destiny. Clinical studies have shown that meditation, when routinely practiced, has important positive effects in the lives of people with back pain. It seems that meditation can help when all else does not seem to work. And, if this is a course you pursue on your own, the financial costs are minimal—it will cost you only the time that you would have spent running around doing tasks you won't remember having done a year from now anyway. What have you got to lose? Perhaps it's time you tried meditation.

Forms Of Meditation

The principle challenge to a person with back pain seeking to meditate is the nearly universal instruction that meditation is best accomplished in a sitting posture. Rather, it's most important that the posture adopted for meditation should be pain-free or provoke pain to the least extent possible. The first key, then, is to adopt a posture that will minimize your back pain; most often this is a lying posture. It is ideal to strive to keep the two sides of the body as symmetrical as possible when meditating. Find a position to meditate in which you will be comfortable for 20–30 minutes. This may mean lying on your back or propping your legs on a sofa, chair, or some pillows as you are lying on your back. Make sure that there are no pressure points underneath you. Lying on a surface that is too firm will provoke inflammation and pain in the body's protective fat pads over the back. When lying on the back, make sure the head is comfortably supported. Most often this will require a pillow that raises the head by two to three inches (5 to 8 cm). Try to meditate at a time when you are not sleepy, but it is okay to feel drowsy, especially if you are taking medicine for pain or if your pain has disrupted nighttime sleeping. Now place your arms at your side or across your body comfortably, take some cleansing breaths, and you are ready to begin!

MUSCLE RELAXATION MEDITATION (PROGRESSIVE RELAXATION)

The technique of purposeful relaxation of various muscles of the body was formalized and promoted by Edmond Jacobson, who worked in this area from the 1920s through the 1960s. The method begins with attention on the feet. By focusing intention on the muscles of the feet, first tense those muscles and then relax them. Attention next moves to the lower part of both legs and the mind focuses on tightening and then relaxing the muscles there. Slowly, calmly breathing in and out and relaxing the muscles of the lower leg more and more fully. Attention then proceeds to the upper leg and onward part by part. The meditation can proceed more or less slowly up the body depending on the progress of the relaxation. If the relaxation is not full enough, more time should be spent on each part and attention should be turned to smaller and smaller parts until the relaxation is successful. A large analysis of clinical studies for back pain showed that progressive relaxation had a large positive effect in terms of reducing back pain.[5]

MANTRA-GUIDED MEDITATION

A widely known form of meditation involves the use of a mantra or simple sound that is repeated over and over to serve as a focal point for the mind. Mantra-guided meditation arises from the Buddhist tradition and has a long and rich heritage.

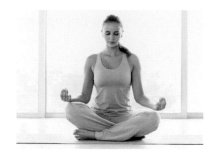

▲ Seated meditation position

ENERGY-BASED OR CHAKRA-CENTERED MEDITATION

Chakra meditation is an offspring of hatha yoga and is a sequential meditation that focuses attention on various centers in the body. These body centers are associated with certain forms of personal energy and with various colors. The Chakra meditation begins by focusing attention at the tail-bone region of the spine, where the associated energy is of being grounded and the color is a dark ruby red. The next Chakra center is in the pelvis, where the energy is creative and the color is tangerine. The third chakra lies in the mid-abdomen over the solar plexus, and has an energy of power and strength and a color of sunshine yellow. The fourth chakra is the heart chakra, which lies in the mid-chest. The associated energy is love and the color is bright green. The fifth chakra is centered in the throat, with energy that promotes effective communication and a color of green-blue. The mind's eye chakra is centered between the eyebrows, and the energy here is foresight. The associated color is deep blue. The seventh and final chakra radiates from the top of the skull, with a transcendent, spiritual energy that is between purple and magenta. The meditation progresses by moving from the first energy center to the seventh, focusing on each one in turn. Several breaths are taken for each chakra. As the breath moves deeply in and out, the mind is brought to focus simultaneously on the location of the Chakra, a visualization of its color, and a contemplation of the value or particular energy associated with each. The purpose of this sequential meditation is to bring the Chakras into appropriate alignment and to leave the meditation practitioner in a state of balance. It is important with this meditation to keep the two halves of the body and mind equally activated.

225

GUIDED IMAGERY MEDITATION

Guided imagery meditation is especially effective for those who are new to meditation, for the very young, and for those who may not be as open to meditation *per se*. Guided imagery may be incorporated into meditation sequences along with other elements such as relaxation and breath-centering. The basic process of guided imagery is to start out with a plan that will walk the mind through a series of events or a journey. The imagery should focus on relaxing events such as a trip to a warm sunny beach, a walk in the park, or a visit to someone you love. For a beach meditation, imagine the feelings of the hot sun as it warms the surroundings and a salty breeze blowing gently over the dunes from the shore. Focus on the soft crunching sound of sand underfoot or a louder sound of people walking on a boardwalk. The sounds of the ocean can be heard in the soft crashing of the waves and the familiar seagull overhead. Focus on sensations that are familiar and comforting. With visualization, it is possible to anticipate challenges and successfully resolve them. It can become a method for tapping into inner strength and solving problems before they occur.

PAIN-DISSOLVING MEDITATION

Although pain-dissolving meditation has evolved independently by pain suffers in response to pain they feel they cannot otherwise control, there is a tradition of meditation that acknowledges pain dissolution as a stage (Vipassana meditation). The core tenet is that intense meditation leads one's mind to eventually let go of the pain. The meditation is actively directed to the site of pain, and seeks to use the mind's powers to dissolve, dilute, or dissipate the pain.

The basics of this approach are fairly straightforward. The meditation begins by finding a quiet space in which one can get into a position of maximum possible comfort. After taking some cleansing breaths, the mind should be directed to the part of the body that is experiencing pain. The mind should be fully concentrated on this body part and the sensations—painful and otherwise—that are arising from that area. Slowly concentrate on seeking out the center of the pain. It may be necessary to creep in from the edges of the pain or possible to zero in immediately. Slowly envision that you are taking this pain and spreading it over the entire body. As it spreads out, it diminishes in intensity almost as waves lapping at the shore will spread out, become paper thin, and then vanish as the tide pulls back. Continue to go into the pain and allow it to extend outward until the strength of your whole body absorbs and dilutes its effects. Don't be discouraged if there is a brief worsening of the pain intensity. Remain aware of the other sensations that are arising from your painful body part. Celebrate those normal non-painful sensations and allow them to grow. Eventually, you will find yourself working at the center of the pain. You may be able to absorb it into the whole of your body and suspend it, if only briefly.

Pain-dissolving meditation requires a lot attention. In most cases, you will need to focus exclusively on this meditation and won't be able to do anything else. And although there are times when a pain flare-up is completely resolved with a single pain-dissolving meditation session (e.g., migraine), it is also the case that pain returns once the meditation is complete. Nonetheless, this is an important pain-relieving technique to learn about and practice.

VALUE-CENTERED (CONCEPT-FOCUSED) MEDITATION

This meditation category encompasses a wide variety of meditations. Your meditation may focus on values such as loving-kindness, compassion, forgiveness, resilience, or non-violence (Ahimsa). This meditation follows the basic principles of finding a comfortable, quiet place to meditate and arranging your schedule so that you can meditate for 25–45 minutes without falling asleep or being rushed away. Some people will approach concept-centered meditation by only allowing the concept itself to be focused upon. Others have recommended an approach in which you allow instances of the concept's opposite to arise into your consciousness as you visualize the events and meditate on how a stronger influence of the desired value would resolve the conflict or problem. This form of meditation may be especially powerful for people who are strongly value-oriented and those who feel that a particular value is under-expressed in their daily lives.

MINDFULNESS MEDITATION FOCUSES ON THE PRESENT

Mindfulness meditation has its origins in Buddhist practice and includes three essential elements: "observe precisely, have equanimity, and be sensitive to how things change."[6] As widely conceptualized and developed in the late twentieth century, however, mindfulness meditation is a non-religious intervention that has been shown to be especially effective for the control of chronic pain.[7] The process of mindfulness meditation includes a body scan meditation, a hatha yoga meditation, and a breath-centered (prana) meditation. The body scan meditation focuses attention on each body part in turn, breathing into that part of the body with the breath in and "feeling" that part of the body dissolve with the breath out. The body scan meditation is intended to bring the practitioner to a state of acceptance or non-striving.

A Bridge to Pain Relief

Although the traditional Eastern approaches to meditation recommend the avoidance of chemical substances, the pain-dissolving meditation described here is an excellent way to engage your mind while waiting for your "rescue medication" to take effect. It is well established that most pain medications require 20 or more minutes to pass before pain relief is perceived. This waiting period can be unbearably difficult sometimes, and knowing that you can use the pain-dissolving meditation to bridge this period and possibly even enhance the effects of the medication is important.

The medical benefits of mindfulness meditation are well established and have even been shown in clinical trials. In fact, the benefits of mindfulness meditation have been specifically proven helpful for back pain. In one study, a group of older adults was offered an eight-week-long mindfulness meditation course for the purpose of improving low back pain.[8] The results were impressive: the patients as a group were more active and less impaired due to their pain. The average amount of meditation was just more than 30 minutes per session, four to five times a week!

BREATHE IN ENERGY, BREATHE OUT NEGATIVITY

It is possible to focus on energy any time one is meditating. The flow of energy may be visualized as entering and leaving the body through the feet, through the breath, or through the part of the body that is closest to the ground. Usually, it is best if the energy flows into the body with each breath in, and negative energy is visualized as departing from the body as the breath is exhaled. It is important to use deep breaths that connect deeply into the lowest parts of the abdomen. Start each breath as if it originated from below the belly button and as you slowly breathe in through the nose, gradually feel your chest fill up with air. As the air enters, concentrate on filling up the lowest parts of the chest first and then the middle. The upper part of the chest will be the last to fill with air. Pause for a moment at the end of each inhalation and slowly begin to release the air from your lungs, chest, and body, starting at the top of the chest and gradually lowering down. This type of breathing has been called *Wave breathing* and is helpful for centering the mind, releasing negative tension, and bringing the thoughts to a fresh beginning.[9]

Other Mind/Body Therapies

ALEXANDER TECHNIQUE: MEDITATION OF THE STARS

The Alexander Technique is a comprehensive system of body movement and motor training designed to optimize the functioning of the body and reduce the physical stress of everyday activities. The technique has long held popularity in the world of actors, musicians, and performance artists, among whom closely attuned body awareness is considered essential. The Alexander Technique originated from the discoveries and teachings of F. Matthias Alexander of Australia and London. It is avidly pursued in parts of England and continues to be taught at the Julliard School in New York and by teachers throughout the U.S. Although it is almost always taught through one-on-one lessons, some exercises have been published as the *Liebowitz Procedures*. In these procedures, the practitioner is guided through a series of movements while thinking of key directions that instruct the body to relax in certain areas that ordinarily carry excessive tension.

One place that usually carries excessive muscle tension is the base of the skull. As such, the Alexander Technique instructs the practitioner to relax the neck and skull, allowing the head to float on the spine as through it is being pulled upward and slightly forward by a helium balloon. As Leibowitz wrote: "Let my neck be free, let my head go forward and up, let my torso widen…"[10] In some parts, the student is instructed to relax specific muscle groups and areas of the body in order to attain the desired result. These skills of relaxation are very useful and can help reduce stress and the pain response when medical procedures are required.

The Alexander Technique has been endorsed by many performers as helping to relieve pain associated with rigorous practice schedules and has been shown in clinical trials to provide long-term relief from chronic or recurrent back pain. In one study, six lessons were found to be nearly as effective as twenty-four lessons.[11]

FELDENKRAIS INTEGRATES MOVEMENT AND THOUGHTS

Feldenkrais is a movement-training methodology developed by Moshe Feldenkrais, a judo master and physicist of the twentieth century with an interest in physiology and neurological aspects of function. The approach is designed to re-teach the body to move more intuitively, and in so doing make the movements of everyday life less stressful. The philosophy of the movement's founder notes that the self consists of movements, sensations, feelings, and thoughts, and that the unfolding of the true self occurs through the conscious alignment of these elements.[12] You can learn the Feldenkrais method through classes or private lessons that teach a series of movements or exercises. The objective of this training is to learn how to function more fluidly and fully with less chance of harm to the body.

Anat Baniel has written a book that brings together some of the physical movements of Feldenkrais technique with a beautiful reorientation towards developing improved vitality in daily life.[13] It is called *Move into Life*. Although it is widely acknowledged that Feldenkrais can be beneficial to those with back pain, one technique in particular is likely to be helpful to those with sacroiliac pain. Loosely described as a variation on the butterfly stretch, the exercise has the student perform a variety of butterfly stretches while sitting upright and lying down. The exercise is entitled *Unexpected Freedom* because of the effect that it has on freeing up the hip joints. It is essential to follow the procedures closely, so borrowing or buying the book will be necessary. The exercises seem to take advantage of normal pressures arising from rocking movements of the legs, hips, and sacrum to gently coax the sacroiliac joint back into position, increasing mobility and potentially reducing pain. Even if you don't suffer with SI joint pain, these exercises are likely to improve the stability of your stance and your flexibility.

229

How to Do Qi Gong's Spinal Breathing

One practice from Qi Gong that is especially helpful for someone recovery from back pain is called *spinal breathing*. To begin, first stand with the feet a wide shoulder-width apart. Holding a good pelvic neutral stance, bend the knees slightly, keeping the tail tucked and the spine upright. Position your arms so they stick straight out from the shoulders with hands facing forward, then bend the elbows to a right angle and make a soft fist with the hands. Now, as you exhale, bring the arms forward and down in front as you flex the spine forward and lower your chin; at the end of your full exhale you should almost be in a standing fetal position. As you begin to breath in, uncurl the spine and bring the arms (still bent) through the starting position and move towards extending the spine as you tilt the chin upwards and the head gently back. At the end of the inhale, you will feel your chest fully expanded as your eyes gaze skywards and your throat and airways fully open. You should feel a good stretch in the chest muscles and a gently distributed tension in the extended back muscles. Do not do this exercise to the point of any pain; this should not hurt in anyway. Repeat the spinal breathing process for a total of eight or more breaths.

QI GONG FOCUSES ON ENERGY FLOW

Qi Gong is sometimes referred to as "moving meditation," designed to promote the flow of energy and clear the mind. As the practitioner of Qi Gong follows the series of movements, they are to focus on the flow of energy into and through the body.[14] Qi Gong is an ancient Eastern practice involving the use of movement and breathing to influence the mind and center the person. Widely practiced and accepted as beneficial by thousands and possibly millions of Eastern practitioners, Qi Gong has been the subject of some political controversy.

As adapted for Western use, Qi Gong is a generally safe and potentially very positive practice. A series of complex movements, Qi Gong practice can help to improve breath awareness, foster a sense of peaceful presence-in-the-moment, and promote overall health consciousness. Qi Gong will help increase your balance and improve lower body strength. Several avenues for learning more about Qi Gong are available. An excellent series of Qi Gong videos has been produced by Lee Holden, and Qi Gong practices are described in books as well.[15]

REIKI TAPS INTO UNIVERSAL ENERGY

Reiki is an energy-based alternative therapy that arose from the work of Mikao Usui in the 1920s.[16] The term *Reiki* is a combination of two words from Japanese, *Rei* and *Ki*, that together mean "universal energy." The process of Reiki involves the placement of hands over or lightly on the fully clothed body with the intention of manipulating the flow of energy. According to Reiki teachings, there are specific patterns of energy in the body that may be in need of healing through the infusion of positive energy.[17] The overall purpose of the therapy is to reduce stress and promote relaxation and healing.

Reiki for the treatment of back pain has not been formally studied, and while smaller-scale studies have not been able to show its specific benefit for conditions such as fibromyalgia, there is evidence to suggest that touch therapies, including Reiki, may be beneficial.[18,19] A recently published study on Reiki for the control of stress and bodily symptoms had a surprising result.[20] It found a benefit to participants who were unaware that the treatment was occurring!

SELF-HYPNOSIS

Hypnosis has been widely used, abused, and disparaged over the centuries. Despite this, there continue to be very helpful applications of hypnosis. Hypnosis is used successfully by pediatricians and pediatric anesthesiologists to relieve children's anxieties about pain and procedures. This is believed to work well because children are much more fluid in their sense of reality and their openness to suggestion. Nonetheless, a majority of adults are considered hypnotizable.

Self-hypnosis is a process of training the mind to enter a state of relaxed wakefulness in which awareness of external events is filtered. It has been described as a relaxed state in which access to the subconscious mind is more direct while conscious awareness is more restricted than usual.[21] Legislation in the state of Connecticut defined hypnosis as "an artificially induced altered state of consciousness, characterized by heightened suggestibility and receptivity to direction."[22]

Hypnosis has been used for a variety of health-related concerns including childbirth, smoking cessation, weight loss, and pain management. A very early clinical trial indicated that hypnosis was as effective as relaxation therapy with respect to pain control and resulted in better sleep and less problematic medication usage.[23] Hypnosis (of others) is regulated in some states and not permitted in some places unless practiced by licensed medical professionals. Self-hypnosis is, obviously, a personal choice and is not regulated, per se. There are many resources available for those interested in self-hypnosis. A recently published study, funded by the National Institutes of Health, found that self-hypnosis was effective at reducing pain and anxiety in women undergoing a large-needle biopsy of the breast.[24] If you are curious about self-hypnosis as a treatment for back pain, ask your doctor, explore your options, and consider investing in some audio-recordings of scripted self-hypnosis sessions (just don't listen to them while driving).

The Explanation

While there are many skeptics of mind-body therapies, there are also many people who support them. One recent study of acupuncture suggested that people who derived the most benefit from acupuncture were those who most expected it to have a benefit.[25] Does this mean that acupuncture doesn't work? It may mean that the person who has the strongest intention to receive a benefit from a therapy is able to experience that therapy more positively and recruit the body's natural health mechanisms in response to the treatment. Despite the persistent doubts of some, millions of people have experienced benefit from meditation and related spiritual practices. In the end, even if there are no immediate health benefits that can be proven in stringent clinical trials, if meditation or other mind-body approaches help you make more healthful choices in life, that is a positive outcome.

CHAPTER RESOURCES

1. Barnes, P.M., E. Powell-Griner, K. McFann, and R.L. Nahin. 2004. Complementary and alternative medicine use among adults: United States, 2002. *Adv Data* 343:1-19.

2. Kabat-Zinn, J., L. Lipworth, and R. Burney. 1985. The clinical use of mindfulness meditation for the self-regulation of chronic pain. *J Behav Med* 8 (2): 163-90.

3. Sherman, K.J., et al. 2004. Complementary and alternative medical therapies for chronic low back pain. *BMC Complement Altern Med* 4:9.

4. Boccio, Frank J. *Mindfulness Yoga*. Somerville, MA: Wisdom Publications, 2004.

5. Ostelo, R.W., et al. 2005. Behavioural treatment for chronic low-back pain. *Cochrane Database Syst Rev* 1:CD002014.

6. Young, Shinzen. *Break through Pain*. Boulder, CO: Sounds True, Inc., 2004.

7. Kabat-Zinn, Jon. *Full Catastrophe Living*. London: Piatkus Books, 2007.

8. Morone, N.E., C.M. Greco, and D.K. Weiner. 2008. Mindfulness meditation for the treatment of chronic low back pain in older adults. *Pain* 134 (3): 310-19.

9. Holden, Lee. *7 Minutes of Magic*. New York: Penguin Group, 2007.

10. Leibowitz, Judith and Bill Connington. *The Alexander Technique*. New York: HarperPerennial, 1991.

11. Little, P., et al. 2008. Randomised controlled trial of Alexander technique lessons, exercise, and massage (ATEAM) for chronic and recurrent back pain. *Br J Sports Med* 42 (12): 965-8.

12. Feldenkrais, Moshe. *Awareness Through Movement*. New York: HarperCollins, 1972.

13. Baniel, Anat. *Move Into Life*. New York: Harmony Books, 2009.

14. Tse, Michael. *Qigong for Healing and Relaxation*. New York: St. Martin's Griffin, 2005.

15. Holden, Lee. *7 Minutes of Magic*. New York: Penguin Group, 2007.

16. "Reiki." http://nccam.nih.gov/health/reiki/. Accessed January 3, 2010.

17. Rand, W.L. "How does Reiki work?" http://www.reiki.org. Accessed January 3, 2010.

18. Assefi, N., et al. 2008. Reiki for the treatment of fibromyalgia: A randomized controlled trial. *J Altern Complement Med* 14 (9): 1115-22.

19. So, P.S., Y. Jiang, and Y. Qin. 2008. Touch therapies for pain relief in adults. *Cochrane Database Syst Rev* 4:CD006535.

20. Bowden, D., et al. 2010. A randomised controlled single-blind trial of the effects of Reiki and positive imagery on well-being and salivary cortisol. *Brain Res Bull* 81 (1): 66-72.

21. MacKenzie, Richard. *Self-Change Hypnosis*. Victoria, BC: Trafford Publishing, 2005.

22. Hypnotherapists Union. Summary of State Laws Regarding Hypnosis, http://www.hypnotherapistsunion.org. Accessed January 4, 2010.

23. McCauley, J.D., et al. 1983. Hypnosis compared to relaxation in the outpatient management of chronic low back pain. *Arch Phys Med Rehabil* 64 (11): 548-52.

24. Lang, E.V., et al. 2006. Adjunctive self-hypnotic relaxation for outpatient medical procedures. *Pain* 126 (1-3): 155-64.

25. Kong, J., et al. 2009. An fMRI study on the interaction and dissociation between expectation of pain relief and acupuncture treatment. *Neuroimage* 47 (3): 1066-76

Q & A *with Dr. Murinson*

Why should I try meditation?

The most important reason to try meditation is to gain control over your pain and your life. As Shinzen Young, a master of meditation has written, "The horrible part of chronic pain is that the more it hurts, the more sensitive you become to the pain. Your pain circuits become pain magnifiers, so that even ordinary sensations are experienced as painful." It is through meditation that you will begin to loosen the tangled knot of pain and movement, and move (in stillness) to a better life.

CHAPTER 20

Water and Inversion Therapies for Strengthening and Conditioning

Gravity-reducing therapies provide immediate pain relief, speed healing, and promote healthy alignment of back structures.

the DIAGNOSIS

> Do you sometimes feel that your back is aching with every step?

> Do you wish you could escape the effects of gravity for a while and get back to feeling like your old self?

If your back has been injured and you have bulging, torn, or herniated discs, you are probably living with substantial amounts of pain. Gravity-reducing therapies can provide immediate relief for your back pain. In addition, studies have shown that reversing gravity's pull may speed the healing of injured discs; help distorted discs and other back structures return to their normal shape; and provide more space for nerves and spinal cord as these delicate structures transit through narrow passages in the back.

In the upright configuration, the spine is under constant pressure. It's clear that standing and sitting up put substantial pressures on the discs, especially in the lower back. This is why people with lumbar disc tears get so much pain relief from lying down. When you're in the water, you are nearly weightless, and this will provide respite for the spine. When you are on an inversion table, the upper part of your body actually creates some mild traction on the lower spine. This process may actually help correct bulging discs and relax tightened muscles.

Listen to Your Body

Maybe you've had the feeling that your back is a little better when you're on vacation, but you haven't wanted to tell people in case they would think your pain is all in your head. It doesn't mean that at all, it just means your body is trying to tell you something about your life, and the message is: It's too much, slow down!

WHAT IF YOUR DOCTOR RECOMMENDS AQUATHERAPY?

Feel good that you have such an open-minded healthcare provider and ask for a prescription. Some insurance companies will cover supervised aquatherapy if prescribed by a physician. If prescription aquatherapy is not what your doctor has in mind, ask about specific programs, frequency, and duration of workouts, and whether the aquatherapy is being recommended as part of a cardiovascular fitness program or your back-strengthening program. There are also online, print, and media-based resources to help with designing a sound water-fitness program.

WHAT IF YOUR DOCTOR RECOMMENDS INVERSION THERAPY?

Ask your doctor what he or she knows about this treatment and how he or she came to recommend it. The clinical trials on inversion therapy are limited, but there is a wealth of testimonials that attest to the benefits of this approach. Ask your doctor to write a prescription for an inversion table or to complete the paperwork to support this recommendation. Some Health Savings Accounts will reimburse you for the purchase of a table if it's done on the advice of a doctor.

the PRESCRIPTION

Gravity-reducing therapies will largely be self-directed, although you should discuss them with your doctor to see if he or she has specific recommendations for aquatherapy or the use of an inversion table.

- Find out about pools in your area. There is no better way to relieve stress on the back than to spend some time in the water. Especially if back pain is preventing you from getting the exercise you need and crave, look into water aerobics, take some swimming lessons, or slip on a water belt and take the plunge.

- If you are truly uncomfortable going to a public or private swimming pool, think about spending a few minutes every day in your bathtub. Of course, it's not possible to get aerobic exercise in the bathtub, but you can benefit from muscle relaxation and minimizing the effects of gravity on the spine.

- Find an aquatherapy specialist in your area and attend a few sessions. Some medical insurers or healthcare reimbursement programs will cover aquatherapy-related expenses if the treatment is prescribed by your doctor.

- While on land, make sure you're getting rest several times daily. This will temporarily stop gravity's effects on your back. The details are in Chapter 13, but you can start by lying down flat on the floor with your legs propped up on a sofa. If you want to reverse the effects of gravity, a slant-board can be a gentle way to get started.

- Consider trying an inversion table. Check in with your local gym to see if it has these available. Long popular with athletic-types, inversion table therapy *may not be for everyone*. But, if you are in pretty good physical shape and want to maximize your at-home therapy for back pain, an inversion table may be right for you. Check with your doctor and start gradually.

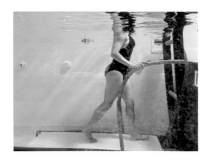

▲ An underwater treadmill used in water-based physical therapy

The Treatment

Water therapy and inversion therapy counteract the effects of gravity on your back. Have you noticed that you are quite a bit shorter in the evening than you are in the morning? Most of us are. Try this: Next time you get into your car, check to see if you have to adjust the mirror up or down. Chances are you adjust the mirror up in the morning and down every afternoon. Over the years, we gradually lose some of our height, although dramatic losses are only typical of diseases such as osteoporosis and ankylosing spondylitis.

Water-Based Therapies

Our bodies are 70 percent water. The rest of our bodies are made up of other things like proteins, minerals (bone), and lipids (fat). To the extent that people have a lot of lipids in their body, they are lighter than water and will be very buoyant. Someone who is very lean will be relatively heavy in water, but even still will feel 70 percent lighter. How can you tell how much body fat you might be carrying around? The National Heart, Lung, and Blood Institute states that "Body mass index (BMI) is a measure of body fat based on height and weight that applies to both adult men and women."[1] You can learn more and check out your BMI numbers in Chapter 21.

If you have a typical body build, meaning you aren't super-athletic or super-sedentary, and you are a middle-aged *man*, your BMI is a fair approximation of your percent body fat.[2] Women should add about 11 percent to the BMI to estimate percent body fat by virtue of our different physiology. The bad news is you may have a lot more body fat than you realized. The good news is that fat floats, and buoyancy will work to your advantage in the water. So as you enter the water, you will feel the weight draining away from your body, you will feel light and relaxed as you float around. If you wear a floatation belt, this will make it easier to keep yourself upright but you won't get as much exercise just staying afloat. In some places, weights are added to the ankles to produce some gentle traction on the spine. However, you don't want to do anything that might jeopardize your ability to keep your head above water. It is wise to always swim in a supervised setting or with someone you know.

WATER WALKING

The exercise that you get from water walking depends on the vigor you apply to it. Water walking can be a gentle and soothing way to remobilize after a painful back injury. As you progress, water walking can become more demanding and even get you going with some cardiovascular fitness.[3] You may want to change your approach from time to time by putting on a flotation belt and doing some water jogging. In water jogging, you are suspended in the water, and as you float you move your legs as if jogging. It's essentially a vigorous form of treading water. Make sure to seek out advice on water walking; there are DVDs and books available.

WATER AEROBICS

This is a wonderful way to maintain and improve physical fitness for people with current or resolved back troubles. The best way to pick up water aerobics is to join a class. In some areas though, water aerobics is the domain of senior citizens, and this may or may not be the best fit. Ask if you can visit a class before signing up. You can check out some books at your library if there are no classes near to your home.[4]

You will want to have access to some special equipment to facilitate your water aerobics workout. A flotation belt will boost your comfort and confidence in the water by allowing you to concentrate on your exercise routine and get your muscles working. Water barbells are not heavy, but work by increasing the drag on your arms as they move through the water. One wonderful aspect of water aerobics is that you are building muscle as you move in both directions, whereas on land, you are usually only building muscle as you move against gravity. Swim gloves can add resistance to your hand movements but are used in place of dumbbells, and flippers may build strength but should not be used during an acute episode of back pain as they may increase strain on the lower back.

WATER STRETCHING AND YOGA

You can use the buoyancy that you gain in water to great advantage in stretching.[5] Find a spot along the wall and practice some lunges and partial splits. You will find that you can focus on the stretch and worry less about straining ankles and knees thanks to the weightlessness. To do the water-lunge, stand next to the wall with one hand on the edge of the pool. Put the foot closest to the wall back about 30 inches (76 cm) and bend your other knee gradually until you feel a stretch in the front of your extending hip (the back leg) and the hamstrings of the flexing hip. Try to keep the heel of the back leg planted down if possible. If you can do this

Warning! Stretch Comfortably and Symmetrically

Whenever you do stretches, in the water or on land, try to find a position that is comfortable enough to hold for a count of 30 seconds. Take baby steps if you're recovering from back pain, and always, always make sure to stretch on both sides to keep your movement patterns symmetrical.

239

stretch comfortably, move your front foot further forward and repeat this stretch for 30 seconds each time, three to five times. Then turn around and stretch the other side.

WATER RELAXATION

This is a wonderful way to end any trip to the pool. Simply find a quiet spot and lie back. Let you body relax as you feel the waves of the pool gently flexing and extending your spine. Close your eyes and empty your mind of worrying thoughts and troubles. You can consciously direct relaxation to your back muscles or just let go and feel at one with the water. Don't rush, just let you body absorb the benefits of your trip to the pool.

Inversion Therapies

Although traction has been widely used for the treatment of back and neck problems, the use of inversion therapies has been relatively slow to gain widespread acceptance in the mainstream medical community. However, inversion therapies have long been popular with fitness buffs and yoga experts. Those who subscribe to inversion therapy tout wide-ranging health benefits, but this is not the objective here; the reason to consider inversion therapy as part of a back-health lifestyle is to ease the pressures on the back and to even begin to reverse the effects of gravity.

Inversion tables offer the widest range of flexibility in terms of being able to control the angle of inversion. You can begin (and continue) with a mild downward tilt of the head. Some inversion tables allow you to set the maximum angle of incline. Others prefer full, hanging-upside-down inversions, and for this, you either need some kind of bar or trapeze arrangement or your need an inversion table. For people of ordinary fitness levels, getting suspended from a bar is not entirely feasible.

Besides the health restrictions on using inversion tables, as noted above, they do require an up-front investment. Even a basic inversion tables is relatively expensive, costing $200 or more, and more sophisticated models range into several hundred dollars. It is not clear why inversion tables have not received more formal testing from the medical community. It could be that inversion tables simply don't work. It could also be that the economics of inversion tables aren't optimal for our healthcare system: they cost just enough to prohibit individuals from wanting to buy them and not enough to be attractive to providers as part of a fee-basis treatment program. Nonetheless, there are many people that really believe that inversion therapy has radically improved their quality of life and taken away most of their back pain. The rationale for this seems sound, but the tables themselves will require further testing before the medical community will accept and promote this treatment.

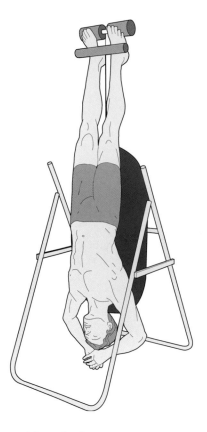

▲ Inversion therapy

SLANT BOARD, A COST-EFFECTIVE METHOD

A slant board is a less expensive alternative to an inversion table that offers some of the benefits, but also some challenges in terms of getting up and down from the partial-inversion position. For many, a slant board is a fitness item designed to increase the amount of work associated with abdominal crunches. It is intended that the user will hook his or her legs over the bars and that the upper body will lie on the negative incline of the board. Depending on the condition of your knees and over all physical condition, this may not sound very restful.

The goal of resting on the slant board is to get the pelvis into a neutral position (hence the need to support the feet) and to let gravity assist in stretching out the spine and muscles. Besides making sure that your slant board arrangement is stable, the real problem is getting on and off the board. If you have an acute disc or acutely painful back problem, it is not a trivial exercise to get yourself positioned on a slant board. If you try to get onto the slant board from a sitting position, you may actually experience some strong pressures on the disc while getting into position. If your back is acutely painful, you may have to lie down on the floor next to the board and slowly scoot yourself up the slope of the board.

Once in position, remember that you need a two-to-three-inch support for your head to make the neck comfortable. You should avoid sliding down the board and pressing on the top of the head, as this can create loading pressure on the spine, especially in the neck.

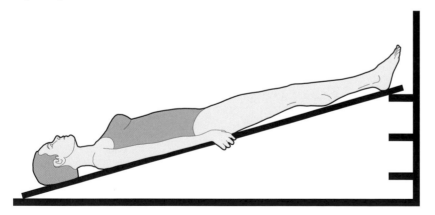

▲ Slant board

Warning! Inversion Therapy Is Not for All

First, it is important that your general health is good. People with heart conditions, high blood pressure, a history of blood clots, problems with circulation such as swelling of the leg, and breathing difficulties should not consider inversion therapies without prior clearance by a qualified physician. If you have particular concerns about trying inversion therapy, a safe alternative might be to try a "zero-gravity" chair.

Do-it-Yourself Slant Board

It's possible to set up a slant board at home using a sturdy support, a solid board, a good foam cushion, and some pillows. You can actually create an arrangement whereby you position your head and spine on a negative incline and have a place that will support your feet as you flex your hips and knees.

INVERTED YOGA POSES

Some yoga poses take advantage of gravity, especially the downward dog. There is a less widely used yoga position called the *hanging dog* that has been adopted by some to involve hanging over various stationary objects.[6] It may be beneficial to suspend yourself upside down from a chair in a supported headstand configuration, but it also may not; you'll have to experiment and see if you can find relief from back pain this way.

The Explanation

Humans enjoy tremendous benefits by virtue of standing on two feet, but, as you look around at other members of the animal kingdom, one curious fact becomes clear. Although myriad creatures from dinosaurs to goldfish follow the same basic outline of having boney spine running through the middle of the body, we are virtually alone in turning this spine upright. This means that gravity is constantly working against us. The problem is most acute in the lumbar spine, where the discs and other spine structures must bear the weight of the upper body. But the cervical spine is also compressed by gravity due to the weight of the head, and this can worsen compression of nerve roots by bulging discs and bone spurs on the spine.[7]

It has been shown by applying traction to the body that unloading the pressures of the lower back can correct disc abnormalities and relieve pain.[8] One study that looked at the effects of traction using serial CT scans of the spine found that traction could reduce the size of disc herniations by 25 percent and increase the space available for nerves exiting the spinal canal by another 25 percent.[9] Traction may be prescribed for your back problem, applied to you by a physical therapist, or used by a chiropractor, but you can apply the basic principles of traction to your advantage using water-based therapies to neutralize gravity or inversion therapy to partially reverse effects of gravity.

CHAPTER RESOURCES

1. NHLBI. "Body Mass Index," www.nhlbisupport.com/bmi. Accessed January 10, 2010.

2. Deurenberg, P., J.A. Weststrate, and J.C. Seidell. 1991. Body mass index as a measure of body fatness: Age- and sex-specific prediction formulas. *Br J Nutr* 65 (2): 105-14.

3. Huey, Lynda and Robert Forster. *The Complete Waterpower Workout Book*. New York: Random House, Inc., 1993.

4. Pappas Baun, MaryBeth. *Fantastic Water Workouts*. Champaign, IL: Human Kinetics, 2008.

5. Huey, Lynda and Robert Forster. *The Complete Waterpower Workout Book*. New York: Random House, Inc., 1993.

6. Levin-Gervasi, Stephanie. *The Back Pain Sourcebook*. Lincolnwood, IL: Lowell House, 1998.

7. Takasaki, H., T. Hall, G. Jull, S. Kaneko, T. Iizawa, and Y. Ikemoto. 2009. The influence of cervical traction, compression, and spurling test on cervical intervertebral foramen size. *Spine (Phila, Pa. 1976)* 34 (16): 1658-62.

8. Horseman, I. and M.W. Morningstar. 2008. Radiographic disk height increase after a trial of multimodal spine rehabilitation and vibration traction: A retrospective case series. *J Chiropr Med* 7 (4): 140-145.

9. Sari, H., U. Akarirmak, I. Karacan, and H. Akman. 2005. Computed tomographic evaluation of lumbar spinal structures during traction. *Physiother Theory Pract* 21 (1): 3-11.

CHAPTER 21

Eating Right to Prevent Pain and Promote Recovery

Moderate weight loss and avoiding trigger foods can improve back pain.

> Are you more than 10 pounds (4.5 kg) overweight?
> Do you eat more than five servings a day of vegetables?
> Do you get gas pains?
> Do you have a burning feeling in your esophagus after meals, or often feel overly full?
> Do you drink eight tall glasses of water a day?
> Do you have a good feeling about any dietary supplements take?

Always include vegetables with the main meals of the day, choose grains that are high in fiber, and seek out calcium, because it is a good defense against worsening spine disease later in life. If you want to eat better for improved back health, read on!

The Treatment

There is no magic food that will cure back pain, but there are a number of positive changes that you can make in your diet to shift the balance toward better back health.

GET A GRIP ON YOUR WEIGHT

Because a lot of back pain is driven by mechanical stresses, how much a person weighs has a profound impact on the back's function. Without question, obesity is a major contributor to back pain and back-related disability. For these reasons, weight control is a priority for those with back pain.

You need to know your numbers. Tomorrow morning, weigh yourself with a reliable scale. Then, get your height measured; you may need help to do this. Have someone make a mark on the doorframe and measure the distance from the floor. You should not have shoes on when measuring your height or weight. You can use the body mass index table in this chapter to find your body mass index (BMI): find your height in the left column of the table; mark this with a highlighter all the way across the table. Follow until you find the number closest to your weight in pounds. Follow this column up to the top row, and this is your BMI number. If your BMI is 24.9 or below, you are in the normal weight category. If your BMI is greater than 25 but less than 29.9, you are in the overweight weight category. If your BMI is 30 or greater, you are obese and should seek medical supervision for a weight-loss plan. If your weight is greater than normal, you should determine the maximum weight you can have to be within normal limits. Do this by following the row for your height until you reach the weight columns for BMI levels of 24 and 25. Your target weight is between these two numbers.

Lasting weight loss can only occur through a combination of decreased food consumption and increased exercise. It is sometimes true that a person can avoid gaining weight by either cutting back on food intake or increasing activity, but true weight loss requires both. If your back is healthy enough that you can engage in cardio-type exercise three times a week, you can realistically plan a new lifestyle that will include reaching a lower target weight. If your back is painful enough that you can't exercise moderately three times weekly, you should not be too hard on yourself if you can't seem to shake excess weight. In fact, for people suffering through an episode of strong back pain, the best, most realistic goal is to avoid weight gain.

BODY MASS INDEX TABLE

BMI	Normal						Overweight				
	19	20	21	22	23	24	25	26	27	28	29
Height in Inches (cm)	Body Weight in Pounds (kg)										
58 (147)	91 (41)	96 (44)	100 (45)	105 (48)	110 (50)	115 (52)	119 (54)	124 (56)	129 (59)	134 (61)	138 (63)
59 (150)	94 (43)	99 (45)	104 (47)	109 (49)	114 (52)	119 (54)	124 (56)	128 (58)	133 (60)	138 (63)	143 (65)
60 (152)	97 (44)	102 (46)	107 (49)	112 (51)	118 (54)	123 (56)	128 (58)	133 (60)	138 (63)	143 (65)	148 (67)
61 (155)	100 (45)	106 (48)	111 (50)	116 (53)	122 (55)	127 (58)	132 (60)	137 (62)	143 (65)	148 (67)	153 (69)
62 (157)	104 (47)	109 (49)	115 (52)	120 (54)	126 (57)	131 (59)	136 (62)	142 (64)	147 (67)	153 (69)	158 (72)
63 (160)	107 (49)	113 (51)	118 (54)	124 (56)	130 (59)	135 (61)	141 (64)	146 (66)	152 (69)	158 (72)	163 (74)
64 (163)	110 (50)	116 (53)	122 (55)	128 (58)	134 (61)	140 (64)	145 (66)	151 (68)	157 (71)	163 (74)	169 (77)
65 (165)	114 (52)	120 (54)	126 (57)	132 (60)	138 (63)	144 (65)	150 (68)	156 (71)	162 (73)	168 (76)	174 (79)
66 (168)	118 (54)	124 (56)	130 (59)	136 (62)	142 (64)	148 (67)	155 (70)	161 (73)	167 (76)	173 (78)	179 (81)
67 (170)	121 (55)	127 (58)	134 (61)	140 (64)	146 (66)	153 (69)	159 (72)	166 (75)	172 (78)	178 (81)	185 (84)
68 (173)	125 (57)	131 (59)	138 (63)	144 (65)	151 (68)	158 (72)	164 (74)	171 (78)	177 (80)	184 (83)	190 (86)
69 (175)	128 (58)	135 (61)	142 (64)	149 (68)	155 (70)	162 (73)	169 (77)	176 (80)	182 (83)	189 (86)	196 (89)
70 (178)	132 (60)	139 (63)	146 (66)	153 (69)	160 (73)	167 (76)	174 (79)	181 (82)	188 (85)	195 (88)	202 (92)
71 (180)	136 (62)	143 (65)	150 (68)	157 (71)	165 (75)	172 (78)	179 (81)	186 (84)	193 (88)	200 (91)	208 (94)
72 (183)	140 (64)	147 (67)	154 (70)	162 (73)	169 (77)	177 (80)	184 (83)	191 (87)	199 (90)	206 (93)	213 (97)
73 (185)	144 (65)	151 (68)	159 (72)	166 (75)	174 (79)	182 (83)	189 (86)	197 (89)	204 (93)	212 (96)	219 (99)
74 (188)	148 (67)	155 (70)	163 (74)	171 (78)	179 (81)	186 (84)	194 (88)	202 (92)	210 (95)	218 (99)	225 (102)
75 (191)	152 (69)	160 (73)	168 (76)	176 (80)	184 (83)	192 (87)	200 (91)	208 (94)	216 (98)	224 (102)	232 (105)
76 (193)	156 (71)	164 (74)	172 (78)	180 (82)	189 (86)	197 (89)	205 (93)	213 (97)	221 (100)	230 (104)	238 (108)

BMI	Obese									
	30	31	32	33	34	35	36	37	38	39
Height in Inches (cm)	Body Weight in Pounds (kg)									
58 (147)	143 (65)	148 (67)	153 (69)	158 (72)	162 (73)	167 (76)	172 (78)	177 (80)	181 (82)	186 (84)
59 (150)	148 (67)	153 (69)	158 (72)	163 (74)	168 (76)	173 (78)	178 (81)	183 (83)	188 (85)	193 (88)
60 (152)	153 (69)	158 (72)	163 (74)	168 (76)	174 (79)	179 (81)	184 (83)	189 (86)	194 (88)	199 (90)
61 (155)	158 (72)	164 (74)	169 (77)	174 (79)	180 (82)	185 (84)	190 (86)	195 (88)	201 (91)	206 (93)
62 (157)	164 (74)	169 (77)	175 (79)	180 (82)	186 (84)	191 (87)	196 (89)	202 (92)	207 (94)	213 (97)
63 (160)	169 (77)	175 (79)	180 (82)	186 (84)	191 (87)	197 (89)	203 (92)	208 (94)	214 (97)	220 (100)
64 (163)	174 (79)	180 (82)	186 (84)	192 (87)	197 (89)	204 (93)	209 (95)	215 (98)	221 (100)	227 (103)
65 (165)	180 (82)	186 (84)	192 (87)	198 (90)	204 (93)	210 (95)	216 (98)	222 (101)	228 (103)	234 (106)
66 (168)	186 (84)	192 (87)	198 (90)	204 (93)	210 (95)	216 (98)	223 (101)	229 (104)	235 (107)	241 (109)
67 (170)	191 (87)	198 (90)	204 (93)	211 (96)	217 (98)	223 (101)	230 (104)	236 (107)	242 (110)	249 (113)
68 (173)	197 (89)	203 (92)	210 (95)	216 (98)	223 (101)	230 (104)	236 (107)	243 (110)	249 (113)	256 (116)
69 (175)	203 (92)	209 (95)	216 (98)	223 (101)	230 (104)	236 (107)	243 (110)	250 (113)	257 (117)	263 (119)
70 (178)	209 (95)	216 (98)	222 (101)	229 (104)	236 (107)	243 (110)	250 (113)	257 (117)	264 (120)	271 (123)
71 (180)	215 (98)	222 (101)	229 (104)	236 (107)	243 (110)	250 (113)	257 (117)	265 (120)	272 (123)	279 (127)
72 (183)	221 (100)	228 (103)	235 (107)	242 (110)	250 (113)	258 (117)	265 (120)	272 (123)	279 (127)	287 (130)
73 (185)	227 (103)	235 (107)	242 (110)	250 (113)	257 (117)	265 (120)	272 (123)	280 (127)	288 (131)	295 (134)
74 (188)	233 (106)	241 (109)	249 (113)	256 (116)	264 (120)	272 (123)	280 (127)	287 (130)	295 (134)	303 (137)
75 (191)	240 (109)	248 (112)	256 (116)	264 (120)	272 (123)	279 (127)	287 (130)	295 (134)	303 (137)	311 (141)
76 (193)	246 (112)	254 (115)	263 (119)	271 (123)	279 (127)	287 (130)	295 (134)	304 (138)	312 (142)	320 (145)

BMI	Extreme Obese							
	40	41	42	43	44	45	46	47
Height in Inches (cm)	Body Weight in Pounds (kg)							
58 (147)	191 (87)	196 (89)	201 (91)	205 (93)	210 (95)	215 (98)	220 (100)	224 (102)
59 (150)	198 (90)	203 (92)	208 (94)	212 (96)	217 (98)	222 (101)	227 (103)	232 (105)
60 (152)	204 (93)	209 (95)	215 (98)	220 (100)	225 (102)	230 (104)	235 (107)	240 (109)
61 (155)	211 (96)	217 (98)	222 (101)	227 (103)	232 (105)	238 (108)	243 (110)	248 (112)
62 (157)	218 (99)	224 (102)	229 (104)	235 (107)	240 (109)	246 (112)	251 (114)	256 (116)
63 (160)	225 (102)	231 (105)	237 (108)	242 (110)	248 (112)	254 (115)	259 (117)	265 (120)
64 (163)	232 (105)	238 (108)	244 (111)	250 (113)	256 (116)	262 (119)	267 (121)	273 (124)
65 (165)	240 (109)	246 (112)	252 (114)	258 (117)	264 (120)	270 (122)	276 (125)	282 (128)
66 (168)	247 (112)	253 (115)	260 (118)	266 (121)	272 (123)	278 (126)	284 (129)	291 (132)
67 (170)	255 (116)	261 (118)	268 (122)	274 (124)	280 (127)	287 (130)	293 (133)	299 (136)
68 (173)	262 (119)	269 (122)	276 (125)	282 (128)	289 (131)	295 (134)	302 (137)	308 (140)
69 (175)	270 (122)	277 (126)	284 (129)	291 (132)	297 (135)	304 (138)	311 (141)	318 (144)
70 (178)	278 (126)	285 (129)	292 (132)	299 (136)	306 (139)	313 (142)	320 (145)	327 (148)
71 (180)	286 (130)	293 (133)	301 (137)	308 (140)	315 (143)	322 (146)	329 (149)	338 (153)
72 (183)	294 (133)	302 (137)	309 (140)	316 (143)	324 (147)	331 (150)	338 (153)	346 (157)
73 (185)	302 (137)	310 (141)	318 (144)	325 (147)	333 (151)	340 (154)	348 (158)	355 (161)
74 (188)	311 (141)	319 (145)	326 (148)	334 (151)	342 (155)	350 (159)	358 (162)	365 (166)
75 (191)	319 (145)	327 (148)	335 (152)	343 (156)	351 (159)	359 (163)	367 (166)	375 (170)
76 (193)	328 (149)	336 (152)	344 (156)	353 (160)	361 (164)	369 (167)	377 (171)	385 (175)

BMI	Extreme Obese (continued)						
	48	49	50	51	52	53	54
Height in Inches (cm)	Body Weight in Pounds (kg)						
58 (147)	229 (104)	234 (106)	239 (108)	244 (111)	248 (112)	253 (115)	258 (117)
59 (150)	237 (108)	242 (110)	247 (112)	252 (114)	257 (117)	262 (119)	267 (121)
60 (152)	245 (111)	250 (113)	255 (116)	261 (118)	266 (121)	271 (123)	276 (125)
61 (155)	254 (115)	259 (117)	264 (120)	269 (122)	275 (125)	280 (127)	285 (129)
62 (157)	262 (119)	267 (121)	273 (124)	278 (126)	284 (129)	289 (131)	295 (134)
63 (160)	270 (122)	278 (126)	282 (128)	287 (130)	293 (133)	299 (136)	304 (138)
64 (163)	279 (127)	285 (129)	291 (132)	296 (134)	302 (137)	308 (140)	314 (142)
65 (165)	288 (131)	294 (133)	300 (136)	306 (139)	312 (142)	318 (144)	324 (147)
66 (168)	297 (135)	303 (137)	309 (140)	315 (143)	322 (146)	328 (149)	334 (151)
67 (170)	306 (139)	312 (142)	319 (145)	325 (147)	331 (150)	338 (153)	344 (156)
68 (173)	315 (143)	322 (146)	328 (149)	335 (152)	341 (155)	348 (158)	354 (161)
69 (175)	324 (147)	331 (150)	338 (153)	345 (156)	351 (159)	358 (162)	365 (166)
70 (178)	334 (151)	341 (155)	348 (158)	355 (161)	362 (164)	369 (167)	376 (171)
71 (180)	343 (156)	351 (159)	358 (162)	365 (166)	372 (169)	379 (172)	386 (175)
72 (183)	353 (160)	361 (164)	368 (167)	375 (170)	383 (174)	390 (177)	397 (180)
73 (185)	363 (165)	371 (168)	378 (171)	386 (175)	393 (178)	401 (182)	408 (185)
74 (188)	373 (169)	381 (173)	389 (176)	396 (180)	404 (183)	412 (187)	420 (191)
75 (191)	383 (174)	391 (177)	399 (181)	407 (185)	415 (188)	423 (192)	431 (195)
76 (193)	394 (179)	402 (182)	410 (186)	418 (190)	426 (193)	435 (197)	443 (201)

Good Food Sources of Calcium	
Milk, 8 oz (230 g) low-fat	300
Mozzarella cheese, 1.5 oz (43 g)	275
Yogurt, 8 oz (230 g), plain	414
Sardines, canned 3 oz (85 g)	324
Kale, 1 cup (130 g), cooked	94
Orange juice, calcium fortified	200

Source: NIH Calcium Factsheet

WHOLE GRAINS, VEGETABLES, AND CALCIUM

Your diet is an important part of your recovery and prevention plan. Diet plays an important role in preventing or reversing obesity, ensuring lifelong overall health maintenance, and providing adequate stores of calcium for strong bones.

Fiber is an important part of staying healthy. The benefits of a high-fiber diet include the prevention of both constipation and diarrhea, potentially reducing cholesterol, a reduction in cancer risk, and (supposedly) the sensation of fullness. Vegetables are an excellent source of dietary fiber, but fiber supplements can be helpful in reaching daily fiber targets. Choosing whole grains whenever possible has become more attractive with the wide array of high-fiber breads now available. Lightly toasting whole grain breads can make them even more appealing.

Vegetables are the best food that you can include in any meal plan. An excellent source of fiber, vitamins, and minerals, they are the best choice for people who snack and should be a part of daily meal planning. Try to include two or more vegetable servings with the main meal of the day. It is best to avoid frying vegetables, but if you love that extra flavor, try sautéing or grilling them instead. Fried vegetables may taste great, but the extra calories are way too much for the body to handle. Most Americans are suffering from caloric overload, and the consequences have been disastrous for the healthcare system.

The CAPS Diet

Foods to avoid:

C – Caffeine and Chocolate

A – Alcoholic beverages

P – Peppermint

S – Spicy foods

Tomatoes are especially high in acid and should be avoided as well.

The need for calcium is also high. The U.S. government recommends that most adults take in over 1,000 mg a day.[1] Dairy products are an obvious choice for people who can tolerate dairy. An 8 oz (230 g) cup of plain yogurt (no fruit) has just over 400 mg. Other sources include calcium-enhanced orange juice, sardines, or canned salmon. Spinach appears to have high levels of calcium, but it also contains oxalic acid, which binds the calcium and interferes with absorption. Kale is a better alternative as a vegetable source of calcium. Turnip greens have twice as much calcium as kale, but also possess a strong flavor. You may want to consider the use of dietary supplements, discussed later in this chapter.

Green vegetables are an essential part of a healthy diet because in addition to calcium they contain magnesium, iron, and potassium. Eat your greens!

FOODS THAT WORSEN BACK PAIN

You may be wondering what you shouldn't eat to reduce your back pain. There are a couple of dietary changes that may help, chief among which is reducing gas in the digestive tract. Because the intestines and certain structures in the back share common nervous system pathways, abdominal gas can increase the amount of pain perceived as arising from the back.[2] And while some people do not have any pain with abdominal gas, others have a surprising amount of pain. Look over the table and identify foods that might be part of the problem. The best way to test this is to eliminate a suspected food for a week or two and see if the abdominal pains get better.

Spicy food might also enhance back pain through a similar mechanism. Some people experience a strong dull pain in the lower abdomen several hours after consuming foods rich in red hot pepper. Because of the time delay, sometimes this low stomach pain seems unrelated to your diet, but keep it in mind.

CAPS FOODS AFFECT THE STOMACH AND ESOPHAGUS

If all the stress of living through an episode of back pain has your stomach churning, try taking control of your diet with the CAPS plan.[3,4] Some of the CAPS plan foods increase stomach acid production, while others cause a loosening of the closed ring that connects the esophagus and stomach. This closed ring, called the *lower esophageal sphincter*, normally opens to allow food into the stomach and stays closed at all other times. Loosening this closure allows stomach acid to enter the esophagus where it can burn the delicate lining (the stomach's lining is heavily protected against stomach acid). Peppermint is one food that loosens the ring between the esophagus and the stomach, so peppermint should be avoided by

Foods that Cause Gas in the Digestive Tract

Food	Offending Agent	Solutions or Alternatives
Beans	Raffinose (a complex sugar)	1. Try rinsing beans before and after cooking. 2. Add Beano before serving. 3. Switch to non-soluble fiber such as wheat-germ or bran.
Cabbage, broccoli, and Brussels sprouts	Raffinose (a complex sugar)	1. Try rinsing foods before and after cooking. 2. Add Beano before serving. 3. Substitute squash, okra, or sweet peppers.
Milk, cheese, and ice cream	Lactose	1. Try taking a lactase supplement before consuming milk products. 2. Substitute yogurt for milk. 3. Seek out low lactose products such as reduced-lactose milk and Swiss cheese. 4. Use soy milk and buy orange juice with calcium added.
Potatoes, corn, pasta, wheat	Various sugars	1. Try rice. 2. Limit quantities of these foods.
Onions, artichokes, and pears	Fructose	1. Substitute small quantities of garlic or onion essence for chopped onion. 2. Try tart apples instead of pears.
Apples, pears, peaches, plums, and prunes	Sorbitol	1. Sorbitol is also used to sweeten diabetic candies; watch out for this ingredient by reading labels. 2. Consume fruits in moderation: no more than three half-cups a day.
Oat bran, peas, beans, and most fruits	Soluble fiber	1. Oat bran may be helpful to lowering blood cholesterol, and its gas-producing effects lessen with time. 2. Limit quantities of these foods and combine with other foods.

Source: "Gas in the digestive tract," National Digestive Diseases Information Clearinghouse. Accessed December 13, 2009

people with reflux symptoms. There are several mechanisms in place to keep stomach acid at effective levels, however, the stress of back pain and some aspects of managing back pain can weaken some of the body's natural defenses against acid reflux. Make sure to cut back on alcohol, as it promotes esophageal damage from reflux—and doesn't mix with many of the medications used for back pain. The association between smoking and gastro esophageal reflux disease (GERD) is less well established, but it is believed that smoking irritates the esophageal sphincter and should be avoided to reduce GERD.

DRINK EIGHT FULL GLASSES OF WATER

Drinking adequate water is important for a healthy back. While it is possible to drink too much water, getting eight 8 oz (235 ml) glasses of water each day is a good goal. Especially if you are taking an NSAID (ibuprofen, naproxen), you will want to stay well hydrated as the combination of dehydration and NSAIDs can be especially taxing on the kidneys. Don't make the mistake of thinking that soda, sweetened teas, or juice can replace your need for water. Many sugar-sweetened sodas contain so much sugar that they are actually dehydrating to the body. Diet sodas seem to be singularly ineffective at helping people lose weight. Think of all the skinny people you know who drink diet soda; now think of all the heavy people you know who drink diet soda: which list is longer?

The benefits of drinking water are tremendous, from improving oral hygiene to reducing food consumption. Most diet experts recommend limiting water intake at mealtime to a few sips. It seems that drinking water in between meals and especially 20 minutes before mealtimes is a good strategy.

Know Your Supplements

GLUCOSAMINE AND CHONDROITIN SULFATE FOR JOINTS

Glucosamine and chondroitin sulfate is the most commonly used non-nutritive dietary supplement for the treatment of arthritis. Derived from cow's hooves and shark cartilage, glucosamine and chondroitin sulfate are compounds that are normally found in joints. The supplementation of these compounds in the diet is believed to contribute to joint motions that are smooth and relatively painless. There is some scientific evidence to support their use in osteoarthritis of the knee and hip.[5,6] A specific benefit for spine arthritis has not yet been shown.[7]

Additional mechanisms may explain the beneficial effects of the compounds against pain. One possibility is that glucosamine in particular may block the release of signaling factors that drive inflammation, but this has been shown in laboratory studies only.[8] Another possibility, shown in several lab-based studies, it that chondroitin may block the sprouting on pain-sensing nerves, which may help prevent pain after back injury as a normally vigorous sprouting response contributes to extra pain sensitivity.[9] There are no recommended doses for this supplement as it is not a nutritive element. A $12 million NIH-funded study examined the effects of glucosamine 1,500 mg and chondroitin 1,200 mg daily and found no benefit in the main study group; however those patients with more severe pain may have had a benefit from the treatment.[10]

CALCIUM FOR BONES

Calcium is clearly important for bone health. Most Americans are not getting enough calcium, and the consequences are a national epidemic of osteoporosis and pathological fractures. The bones prone to fracture include the vertebral bones, pelvic bones, and hips, all potential sources of severe back and buttock pain. As noted above, the daily requirement for calcium is at least 1,000 mg daily. Most adults have difficulty reaching this goal. The two main forms of calcium supplements available are calcium carbonate and calcium citrate. Calcium carbonate is usually less expensive and more readily available. Calcium citrate is probably better absorbed by people with low levels of stomach acid (those who may be taking medication for GERD/reflux fall into this category). Additionally, it is recommended that the amount taken at any one time during the day is 500 mg, as this will improve overall absorption and limit troublesome side effects such as constipation and bloating that occur at higher doses.

VITAMIN D FOR BONES, NERVES, MUSCLES, AND IMMUNITY

Vitamin D is vitally important for bone health. Without vitamin D, calcium is not properly deposited into bones and bones become thin and fragile. Not getting enough vitamin D can lead to osteoporosis and osteomalacia (severe decalcification of the bones), predisposing to vertebral fracture and ultimately spinal collapse.

The NIH has reported that vitamin D is also involved in the function of nerves, muscles, and the immune system (ODS/NIH). Vitamin D has been shown to reduce inflammation. More controversial are the claims that vitamin D insufficiency is a leading cause of chronic pain. There are a number of studies, summarized by Leavitt, that suggest a possible link between supplementation of vitamin D and a cessation of chronic pain.[11,12] More studies are needed before definitive recommendations can be made; however, many physicians are offering to order testing of vitamin D levels for their patients because of the serious risks of vitamin D deficiency. Factors that contribute to the need for increased dietary intake include decreased levels of sun exposure and the use of sun screens that block UV-B rays. The NIH

Factors That Increase Stomach Acid Reflux

- Stress
- Ibuprofen and other NSAIDs
- Lying down soon after meals
- CAPS foods
- Frequent bending over
- Heavy lifting
- Obesity
- Fatty foods

Special Tips:

- Rinse canned tuna and packaged lunchmeats; this will lower your sodium intake. Avoid canned vegetables; substitute fresh or frozen wherever possible.

- Only buy low-fat milk, or fat-free if you can tolerate the "skim-milk" taste.

- Use only low-fat cheese.

- Use your microwave to cook your vegetables: They come out brighter and tastier than stove-top veggies.

- Make soup once a week in the winter (but get someone to help lift that heavy soup pot off the stove when necessary).

- Grow your own herbs for seasoning: chives, dill, and basil are especially easy to cultivate.

- Make sure to include fish in your diet.

recommends limiting vitamin D intake to no more than 2000 IU daily. Interestingly, the recommended intake of vitamin D increases with age, so while adults under 50 years old are advised to take in 200 international units (IU) a day, adults 50 to 70 should consume 400 IU daily, and adults over 70 should consume 600 IU.

VITAMIN B_{12} FOR MUSCLES AND NERVES

Vitamin B_{12} may help alleviate back pain, as shown in a clinical trial.[13] It is an essential element in the metabolism of muscles and nerves. In conditions of deficiency, people experience depression, bizarre tingling sensations, and often times diffuse, poorly explained pains. The association of B_{12} and back pain is probably limited in younger adults, although it is now believed that B_{12} deficiency is more prevalent than previously thought. The tendency to vitamin B_{12} deficiency increases with age and may exceed 15 percent of the population. There is essentially no upper limit to the consumption of vitamin B_{12}; however, recommended intake levels are relatively small: 2.4 micrograms daily for most adults. Good food sources of vitamin B_{12} include beef liver, trout, salmon, and fortified breakfast cereal.

An important challenge to maintaining normal levels of vitamin B_{12} is that the absorption of this vitamin depends on a protein made in the stomach and also on normal stomach acidity. In many older adults, there is a failure of vitamin B_{12} absorption; as the stomach fails to make the necessary chaperone protein, B_{12} levels in the blood gradually fall and the onset of deficiency is creeping and insidious. A supplement of B_{12} dissolved under the tongue may be an effective replacement for the vitamin shots that have been prescribed in past years; however, this therapy should be implemented under the supervision of your doctor. It seems that many of the medicines used for acid reflux may also interfere with vitamin B_{12} absorption by reducing stomach acid. Talk with your doctor about checking your levels regularly if you are on long-term treatment with these medications.

DIETARY SUPPLEMENTS THAT MIGHT CAUSE HARM

- Vitamin B_6 taken at high doses may actually cause a painful neuropathy. Taking vitamin B_6 at doses significantly above the daily recommendations has been shown to destroy nerves and cause pain. It is prudent not to consume more than 250 percent of the daily recommended amounts of B_6: Add up the percentages from all your vitamins to determine your current intake.

- Excessive intake of the fat-soluble vitamins A, D, E, and K should be avoided. It is difficult for the body to remove any unneeded amounts of these vitamins, and toxic accumulations can occur.

FOODS WITH ANTI-INFLAMMATORY PROPERTIES

Turmeric contains a compound, curcumin, which has been shown in laboratory studies to have activity against molecules that signal inflammation. However, the ability of this compound to enter the blood stream is limited, and the benefits of consuming turmeric as a food or supplement have not been definitively proven.[14]

AVOID PRO-INFLAMMATORY FOODS

Omega-6 oils are precursors to pro-inflammatory compounds in the body, called eicosanoids. Eicosanoids drive inflammatory and pain signals in the body. Omega-6 oils are especially rich in corn, safflower, and sunflower cooking oils. It is better to limit the use of these oils; substitute olive and canola oils.[15]

MORE RESOURCES

While losing weight when you are sidelined by back pain may be impossible, you can vary your diet to help with your back. In this chapter, I've highlighted some possible changes that may be helpful to you in your quest for improved back health. You will find other valuable resources at the American Heart Association, the National Center for Complimentary and Alternative Medicine, the NIH, and the National Digestive Diseases Clearinghouse websites.

CHAPTER RESOURCES

1. NIH. "Calcium Fact Sheet," http://dietarysupplements.info.nih.gov/factsheets/calcium.asp. Accessed January 31, 2010.

2. Gao, J., et al. 2006. Enhanced responses of the anterior cingulate cortex neurones to colonic distension in viscerally hypersensitive rats. *J Physiol* 570: 169-83.

3. Mullick, T., and J. E. Richter. 2000. Chronic GERD: Strategies to relieve symptoms and manage complications. *Geriatrics* 55: 28-43.

4. Kahrilas, P. J. 1996. Gastroesophageal reflux disease. *JAMA* 276: 983-88.

5. Herrero-Beaumont, G., et al. 2007. Glucosamine sulfate in the treatment of knee osteoarthritis symptoms. *Arthritis Rheum* 56 (2): 555-67.

6. Pavelká, K., et al. 2002. Glucosamine sulfate use and delay of progression of knee osteoarthritis. *Arch Intern Med* 162 (18): 2113-23.

7. Leffler, C.T., et al. 1999. Glucosamine, chondroitin, and manganese ascorbate for degenerative joint disease of the knee or low back. *Mil Med* 164 (2): 85-91.

8. Walsh, A.J., C.W. O'Neill, and J.C. Lotz. 2007. Glucosamine HCl alters production of inflammatory mediators by rat intervertebral disc cells in vitro. *Spine J* 7 (5): 601-8.

9. Grimpe, B., et al. 2005. The role of proteoglycans in Schwann cell/astrocyte interactions and in regeneration failure at PNS/CNS interfaces. *Mol Cell Neurosci* 28 (1): 18-29.

10. Clegg, D.O., et al. 2006. Glucosamine, chondroitin sulfate, and the two in combination for painful knee osteoarthritis. *N Engl J Med* 354 (8): 795-808.

11. Leavitt, S.B. "Vitamin D – A Neglected 'Analgesic' for Chronic Musculoskeletal Pain, An Evidence-Based Review and Clinical Practice Guidance." Medical Reviewers Bruce Hollis, Ph.D., Michael F. Holick, M.D., Ph.D., et al. June 2008, http://Pain-Topics.org/VitaminD.

12. Schwalfenberg, G. 2009. Improvement of chronic back pain or failed back surgery with vitamin D repletion: A case series. *JABFM* 22 (1): 69-74.

13. Mauro, G.L., et al. 2000. Vitamin B_{12} in low back pain: A randomised, double-blind, placebo-controlled study. Eur Rev Med *Pharmacol Sci* 4 (3): 53-8.

14. Henrotin, Y., et al. 2010. Biological actions of curcumin on articular chondrocytes. *Osteoarthritis Cartilage* 18 (2): 141-9.

15. Baskette, Michael and Eleanor Mainella. *The Art of Nutritional Cooking, Second Edition*. Upper Saddle River, NJ: Prentice Hall, 1999.

CHAPTER 22

Your Back: A Guided Tour

Know the mechanisms of your back pain.

> Do you ever wonder how you can be hurting so much, but your doctors don't know reason why?

> Why does some pain seem to last forever, while other pain goes away when the wound heals?

Learning about the anatomy of your spine and the physiology of how pain works can help you answer questions such as these. This chapter will take you on a quick tour of the spine and provide a brief description of how your body processes pain.

Anatomy of the Spine

Regardless of size, spines follow a one-design-fits-all biological model, which involves bony structures called vertebrae stacked on top of each other in a canal. Dinosaurs, humans, monkeys, mice, and all related creatures have variations of the same model. Remarkably, they all share the same combination of vertebrae, from delicate structures in the neck to sturdier structures in the lower back. These common characteristics are where we get the name for our species: vertebrates.

There is one major difference in the spines of some vertebrates. Humans and other closely related animals have vertically organized spinal columns and walk on two legs. Most other vertebrates—from big black bears to mice—have horizontally organized spines and walk on all fours. The vertical spine has some advantages. For example, being upright gives us the use of our hands while walking or running, and we are taller than we would be on all fours. The downside is that our upright posture leaves us prone to wear and tear of the discs and related structures of the spine, as well as other problems of the back.

Spines have three curves forming an S shape. They are the cervical, thoracic, and lumbrosacral curves, named for the types of vertebrae they include. Following the S-shaped path, your spine sits in a canal that runs down the length of your back from your brain to your bottom. The spine is made up of bones, ligaments, tendons, large muscles, weight-bearing joints, and highly sensitive nerves. It's the center of control for your posture and provides stability when you stand. It also houses and protects your all-important spinal cord, the communication route for your brain and nervous system. Unfortunately, because the spine has so many tasks, it is highly susceptible to injury, which can strike its vertabrae, ligaments, discs, or muscles. Bone spurs or scar tissue along the spine can also press against nerve roots causing pain.

VERTEBRAE SUPPORT MUSCLES AND ALLOW FOR MOTION

Vertebrae are the box-shaped bones that provide the architecture for your spine and carry most of the weight placed on it. They are formed in part by strong, sturdy, and flexible cancellous (spongy) bone containing a core of marrow, which produces red blood cells. Most adults' spines have 32 vertebrae, stacked on top of each other. The vertebrae meet at joints, which allow for slight movement. Sometimes people have one fewer or one extra vertebra, but this is not mechanically advantageous.

There are five different types of vertebrae:

- Cervical vertebrae: Seven vertebrae that hold up your neck and allow it to move right and left.
- Thoracic vertebrae Two vertebrae that are located in the middle back and extend forward as the ribs. They help protect the heart and lungs and support the weight of the arms and shoulders. Because they are limited in movement, they rarely have herniated discs.
- Lumbar vertebrae: Five vertebrae located in the lower back. They are the largest vertebrae and carry most of your body's weight, which is why so many people have pain in this area. These vertebrae allow forward and backward motion.
- Sacrum: Five vertebrae located below the lumbar vertebrae. They are fused together in one triangular section. The sacrum provides attachment for the hip bones and protects organs.
- Coccyx: Three vertebrae located at the very bottom of the spine. They are also fused. They support the muscles of the buttocks.

FACET JOINTS LINK THE VERTEBRAE

Housed between your vertebrae are structures called *facet joints*. The facets are bony knobs that link the vertebrae together and make it possible for them to move against each other. The facet joints give the spine its flexibility. A smooth lining called the synovium sits between the facet joints. The lining produces synovial fluid, which nourishes and lubricates the joint.

Back Facts: The Spine

- Is the platform for and provides flexibility for your head, which weighs in the neighborhood of 11 pounds (5 kg).

- Supports and provides flexibility for your upper body. Your spine allows you to bend forward, backward, and sideways.

- Provides shelter for and protects your spinal cord and nerves.

- Is one of the key structures in your skeleton, and has many essential muscles and ligaments attached.

THE SPINAL CORD CARRIES CELLS AND NERVES

Part of the central nervous system, your spinal cord is rich with cells and nerve pathways that run about 18 inches (46 cm) from the bottom of your brainstem all the way down to your lower back. Although it plays a leading role in the nervous system, the spinal cord is relatively delicate and small. (It is the width of your little finger.) The spinal cord is protected by the 32 vertebrae of the spine.

Spinal cords have two types of nerves: white matter, which are also called *long tracts* because as nerves go, they are quite long, and grey matter. Long tracts control messages from the brain to distant parts of the body. They don't stop along the way to converse with individual neurons (cells that send electrical signals to other neurons). They also connect different sections of the spinal cord to each other. Grey matter makes connections between individual neurons.

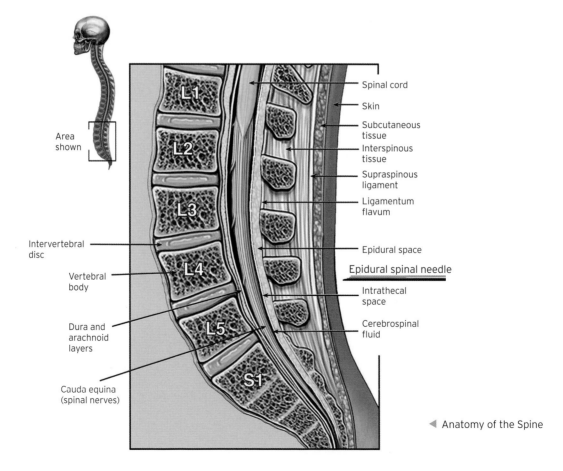

◀ Anatomy of the Spine

THE SPINAL CANAL HOUSES THE SPINAL CORD

The spinal cord sits in the spinal canal. Vertebral bodies form the floor of the canal and flat bones called *lamina* form the roof. Ducts where nerves exit and enter the spine sit on the walls of the canal. Between each wall are supporting structures called pedicles.

DISCS ABSORB SHOCKS

Discs sit between the vertebrae where they serve as spacers and provide cushioning. The discs contain a gel-like fluid called *nucleus pulposus*, which is primarily water.

Vertebrae discs are supported in part by a tough outer layer called the *annulus fibrosis*. Along with the vertebrae, the discs and annulus fibrosis cushion the spine. When pressure occurs, such as when you lift something heavy or twist around, the nucleus pulposus is compressed. When the lifting, twisting, or other activity stops, the gel goes back to its original shape. The vertebrae discs also safeguard the openings where the nerves exit the spinal cord.

Vertebrae discs are often the guilty party behind back pain. The nucleus pulposus can rupture, leaking or bulging out and pressing against nerves that line the spine. The discs in the cervical and lumbar regions are the most likely to rupture. This painful back condition may be a torn disc, herniated disc, slipped disc, ruptured disc, bulging disc, prolapsed disc, or protruding disc.

MUSCLES, TENDONS, AND LIGAMENTS

The muscles running up and down your back support your spine. When these muscles are strong, they also protect your back and help you move around with ease. But if they become weak due to lack of exercise, aging, obesity, or for other reasons, your spine is far less flexible and more easily injured.

The muscles in your stomach area and trunk also help support your spine and aid mobility. In addition, tendons connect your muscles to your bones, and ligaments join your vertebrae together. Ligaments also provide your spine with flexibility and control.

Pain Pathways: A Guided Tour

It is helpful to your understanding of back pain to know how nerve signals leave the site of an injury, travel to your brain, and return as a feeling that hurts. In addition, there are mysterious features of pain that you may encounter and would like to understand better. For example, pain may occur for what appears to be no reason at all. The cause of the pain has long since healed, has probably even been forgotten about, but pain continues, sometimes for a very long time. This is called *neuropathic pain*, and I discuss it and other pain concepts in the following sections.

THE NERVOUS SYSTEM COMMUNICATES PAIN

Your nervous system is your body's communication highway for pain. It has two parts:
- The brain and spinal cord, also known as the central nervous system (CNS).
- The peripheral nervous system (PNS), which includes all the sensory and motor nerves that go to and from your CNS.

NERVE CELLS SEND SIGNALS

Pain is a response to an injury by specific types of nerve cells (neurons) in your PNS called *nociceptors*. Their job is to warn your brain when an injury has occurred. In the case of back pain, the injury may be the result of any harmful event from small to catastrophic, such as a pinched nerve or a car crash. There are four others concepts in the pain process that you should be familiar with:
- *Sensitization* occurs when nerve cells release neurotransmitters that actually increase the strength of the pain messages being sent to your brain.
- *Inflammation* is your body's response from an injury that may result in redness, heat, pain, swelling, and loss of function. It often piles on additional pain in the area surrounding an injury. Inflammation can also be a cause of sensitization.
- *Allodynia* is pain caused by something that does not normally elicit it, such as a brush stroke or bed sheets. Allodynia can accompany many other painful conditions such as neuropathies and severe injuries.
- *Hyperalgesia* is an amplified pain response to an injury that normally would provoke far less pain. In medical terms, this means that the individual's "pain threshold" is reduced. Hyperalgesia can strike a discrete area of the body or be widespread. The condition has three subtypes:
  - *Primary hyperalgesia* is increased pain sensitivity in the damaged tissues.
  - *Secondary hyperalgesia* is increased pain sensitivity in surrounding undamaged tissues.
  - *Opioid-induced hyperalgesia* is increased pain sensitivity caused by long-term opioid (narcotic) use.

Types Of Pain

There are three major types of pain: nociceptive, inflammatory, and neuropathic. All three types of pain are important for back pain: They can co-exist or occur separately. Treatment strategies vary depending on pain type involved.

NOCICEPTIVE PAIN

As the name suggests, nociceptive pain occurs when pain-sensing nerve endings are stimulated by injury or an injurious stimulus. Anything that potentially damages body tissues, such as a blow, a cut, or a burn, can result in nociceptive pain.

INFLAMMATORY PAIN

Inflammatory pain arises from changes in the pain signaling system due to inflammation. When inflammation arises, there is an increase in the local prod-uction of "inflammatory signaling molecules;" these change how sensory signals are processed.

Often, inflammatory pain is characterized by a strong amplification of pain sensation: a mildly painful stimulus gets translated into a stronger, sharper pain. Inflammatory pain can also be characterized by pain in response to a stimulus that is not normally painful, for example gently bumping an ingrown toenail. NSAIDs are usually helpful for inflammatory pain.

NEUROPATHIC PAIN

Neuropathic pain is caused by damage to or malfunction of the body's sensory system. In neuropathic pain, the body's pain sensing system is no longer a faithful reporter of injury. Neuropathic nerves will signal damage where none exists and over-amplify minor insults. The result is a marked increase in pain and suffering. Neuropathic pain can occur after a stroke, spinal cord injury, or diabetes. NSAIDs usually do not help patients with neuropathic pain.

ACUTE VERSUS CHRONIC BACK PAIN

Acute pain leaves when the injury is healed. Chronic pain lingers on, often greatly affecting the quality of life of the patient. Sometimes the culprit behind chronic pain is a health problem such as rheumatoid arthritis, which by definition causes continuing and persistent damage to body tissues and keeps pain pathways busy.

Sometimes the nervous system does not get the message to stop sending pain signals. In other words, it doesn't shut down even though the injury has long since healed. In such cases, the actual cause of the stubborn pain process can be difficult to detect.

Chronic back pain commonly hits (and stays with) you in one of two ways:
- Constant: It's present for more than three months.
- Recurring: The pain stays for long periods of time. Then it leaves only to come back again. This maddening pattern can continue for months or years.

KNOWLEDGE IS POWER FOR YOUR BACK

The pain-sensing system plays a vital role in helping us to protect ourselves from bodily harm. It is a tragic, but valuable lesson to learn that children who are born without an intact pain system are prone to recurrent injuries, and often do not survive to adulthood. Nonetheless, if the sales of pain-medications are any indicator, we collectively have a lot more pain than we are really coping with.

This book was designed to equip you with the knowledge and skills to live a better and healthier life, and "make peace with your back." If the measures described here are not sufficient to get you comfortable and moving again, you'll need to speak with your doctor about surgery or prescription medications. If the recommendation is for medication, it's important to know that there are many, many medications that can be used in the treatment of back pain. Sometimes, these medications work better when used together; sometimes finding a single medication that targets the core of a problem is sufficient. Learn, ask questions, and learn some more. Learning more about your body and your back will only help you navigate this challenging course.

ACKNOWLEDGMENTS

With thanks to Jill Alexander, my senior editor at Fair Winds Press, who has brought this project to happy fruition; to Laura B. Smith, who ran like the wind with this manuscript, infusing positive energy along the way; to the production staff, who gave the book sparkle. To Marilyn Allen, an agent par excellence and a connoisseur of beautiful books.

Many people contributed to the conceptualization and realization of this project: Pamela Talalay, for her indefatigable encouragement and keen wit; Thomas Brushart, who inspired me to write my own book; Justin McArthur, who has at many turns supported my career development; Dick Meyer, Jim Campbell, Jack Griffin, Marco Rizzo, Lew Levy, Steve Waxman, and Bob Kalb for their support of my interest in pain; Dina Adams for lending her expertise in physical therapy and her contributions to the therapeutic plan in earlier versions of this project; Michael Shear for his demonstration that an excellent physician must, as Hippocrates said, be prepared to "make the patient, the attendants, and the externals cooperate."

Thanks to those who have read and provided sage comments on the manuscript: Ann Frontera-Rial, Chaim and Mindy Landau, and Zan Vautrinot. Thanks to my children: Eitan for doing his homework at the table and keeping me company, and Rachel, who has taught me to say "goodnight computer." To Eleanor Mainella, for her careful reading of and guidance that improved the diet chapter. To my mom, Eila Mae, for teaching me to be a happy learner, and to my dad, Donald, who has always believed I could accomplish my dreams. To Sol Milgrome, who taught me to "take a negative and make a positive." And to Sasha, my beloved, for his partnership, encouragement, and kindness in all things.

ABOUT THE AUTHOR

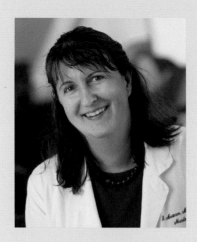

Beth B. Murinson, M.S., M.D., Ph.D., is an attending physician, scientist, and director of pain education in Neurology at the Johns Hopkins School of Medicine, where she also chairs the Pain Management Task Force.

Murinson, a 2001 Diplomate in Neurology, American Board of Neurology and Psychiatry, trained in neurology at Yale University under the direction of Stephen G. Waxman and completed a three-year clinical and research fellowship at Johns Hopkins School of Medicine under the direction of John W. Griffin. She is currently part of a small team of Hopkins neurologists who spend significant clinical time in intraoperative monitoring. In this, she utilizes all electrodiagnostic modalities including electromyography; nerve conduction studies; electroencephalography; sensory, motor, and auditory evoked potentials; and cortical mapping. Murinson has clinical expertise on neuropathic pain and back pain, and she manages patients with both immune-mediated neurological disease as well as chronic pain due to injury or neuro-degenerative disease. Murinson is skilled in performing nerve and muscle biopsies. She has been recognized by peers as an outstanding physician and was selected as one of Baltimore's "Top Doctors" for 2007.

Murinson has an active laboratory research program and has directed the training of numerous students in this context. Her current laboratory research focuses on two questions. The first is a translational science project that examines the origins of drug-induced effects on the peripheral nervous system. Taking a highly novel approach, she has led a team of experts in investigating the effects of widely prescribed drugs on nerves and related cells in culture. The results indicate that pathways related to neurotrophin signaling are likely to mediate these effects. The second is the development of a novel model of neuropathic nerve injury. In this model, Murinson is endeavoring to isolate the effects of neuronal degeneration and better define the role of the intact nerve in signaling the effects of injury. Murinson is the author of more than 20 peer-reviewed publications, as well as numerous book chapters on pain. She is a peer-reviewer for *Annals of Neurology, Neurology,* and *Brain and Nature.*

Murinson is one of a select group of core faculty members committed to medical education and chosen for inclusion in the Johns Hopkins Colleges Advisory and Clinical Skills Program. She leads a multidisciplinary team seeking to understand the emotional development of medical students and how medical trainees learn best about pain. Results of her educational research are published in the *Journal of Pain and Academic Medicine* and have been presented at the American Pain Society and the International Association for the Study of Pain meetings. She has served as co-director of the research program for the 2007 national Learning Communities meeting in conjunction with the AAMC meeting and has served on a Panel for the U.S. National Board of Medical Examiners. Director of a new, clinically-focused curriculum in pain at Johns Hopkins, Murinson is a 2005 Diplomate of the American Board of Pain Medicine.

Murinson is a wife and the mother of two children. She enjoys reading books with her kids and excels at helping with math homework, piano lessons, and art projects.

IMAGE CREDITS

Page 21: originally published in *Yoga Beats the Blues*; page 26: © Universal Images Group Limited / Alamy; page 35: © Nucleus Medical Art, Inc. / Alamy; page 65: MEDICAL RF.COM / SCIENCE PHOTO LIBRARY; page 88: © medicalpicture / Alamy; page 100, top: NEIL BORDEN / SCIENCE PHOTO LIBRARY; page 114: SCOTT CAMAZINE / SCIENCE PHOTO LIBRARY; page 117: © Nucleus Medical Art, Inc. / Alamy; page 127: ALAIN POL, ISM / SCIENCE PHOTO LIBRARY; page 129, top: © Nucleus Medical Art, Inc. / Alamy; page 136, top: LIVING ART ENTERPRISES / SCIENCE PHOTO LIBRARY; page 136, bottom: LIVING ART ENTERPRISES / SCIENCE PHOTO LIBRARY; page 137: DU CANE MEDICAL IMAGING LTD / SCIENCE PHOTO LIBRARY; page 146: © Sebastian Kaulitzki / Alamy; page 153: © Nucleus Medical Art, Inc. / Alamy; page 163, top: BO VEISLAND / SCIENCE PHOTO LIBRARY; page 182: originally published in *Tamilee Webb's Defy Gravity Workout*; page 183: originally published in Yoga *Turns Back the Clock*; page 184: originally published in *Yoga Turns Back the Clock*; page 186: originally published in *Yoga Turns Back the Clock*; page 224: Tony Hutchings / Getty Images; page 225: istockphoto.com; page 238: istock-photo.com; page 260: © Nucleus Medical Art, Inc. / Alamy

INDEX